The Grace of Forgetting:
A Joyful Reimagining
of Alzheimer's
and Memory Loss

The Grace of Forgetting: A Joyful Reimagining of Alzheimer's and Memory Loss

Francis Williams

To Rachael and Nathanael

My Candles in the dark,
when the lights go out.

Copyright Page

Copyright © 2025 by Francis Williams

All rights reserved.

Title: The Grace of Forgetting:
A Joyful Reimagining of Alzheimer's and Memory Loss

Author: Francis Williams

Publisher: Quite Frank Educational Services
Richmond, BC, Canada

Cover Design: By the author
Printed in the United States of America

ISBN: 978-1-997668-40-4

The Grace of Forgetting:
A Joyful Reimagining of Alzheimer's
and Memory Loss
Francis Williams

Table of Contents

Disclaimer and Acknowledgment

This book is intended for informational, reflective, and emotional support purposes only. It is not a substitute for professional medical advice, diagnosis, or treatment. Always seek the guidance of qualified health professionals or licensed therapists with any questions you may have regarding dementia, Alzheimer's disease, or caregiving practices. Never disregard professional advice or delay seeking it because of something you have read in this book.

Every individual's experience with memory loss is unique, and while the insights offered here may be helpful or illuminating, they may not apply to every situation. The content in this book is not intended to offer clinical or legal recommendations, nor is it meant to represent the views of any specific institution or organization.

AI Tools and Creative Collaboration

This book was developed with the support of advanced artificial intelligence tools, which were used for:

- Research aggregation
- Drafting, editing, and structuring content
- Synthesizing philosophical and cultural frameworks
- Generating creative language and narrative flow

The use of AI in the writing process enabled a more expansive and integrated exploration of Alzheimer's and memory loss through a compassionate and reimagined lens. All AI-generated content was curated, reviewed, and shaped with intentional human oversight to ensure accuracy, emotional resonance, and ethical integrity.

We acknowledge that the use of AI is an evolving practice and recognize the importance of transparency in its role in the creative process.

The heart of this book, however, comes from real human experiences—those of caregivers, families, friends, and individuals living through the complexities of memory loss with grace, struggle, and love. AI served as a tool, but the spirit of the work is human.

Introduction

The Grace of Forgetting: A Joyful Reimagining of Alzheimer's and Memory Loss

Alzheimer's disease and memory loss are often portrayed in the Western world as unrelenting tragedies—a slow erasure of self, a long goodbye. Families brace for grief long before death. Words like "devastating," "heartbreaking," and "hopeless" dominate the conversation. We talk about "losing" our loved ones even while they are still with us. The overwhelming narrative is one of fear, sorrow, and inevitable decline.

But what if there is another story waiting to be told? One rooted not in denial or sugarcoating, but in presence, joy, and liberation. What if letting go of memory is not just a loss, but also a release—a return to essence? What if the slow unwinding of identity offers a different kind of freedom, both for the person experiencing it and for those who love them?

This book is a radical reframing. It invites you to step out of the cultural assumptions that surround Alzheimer's and other forms of dementia and to consider a more compassionate, connected, and joyful approach. Not because memory loss is easy—it isn't—but because we are not bound to one narrative of suffering. We can choose to see beauty in the fragments, to laugh at what we once feared, to meet one another in the moment, again and again.

In Western culture, we prize intellect and continuity of self. We hold tight to our personal stories, our achievements, our memories, our names. When those things begin to slip away, we panic. We interpret it as the unraveling of the soul. But many other cultures see identity differently. In Buddhist teachings, for example, the self is already an illusion—a construct of the mind that's always changing. In Indigenous traditions, being is often relational, not individual. In spiritual mysticism, surrender

1

is not a loss but a pathway to unity. What if we let those perspectives help shape how we understand memory loss?

Alzheimer's, in this light, can become something else entirely. It can be a passage into the present moment, where love does not depend on words or history. It can be a dance of attention and acceptance. It can invite families to slow down, simplify, and communicate with the heart instead of the head. It can be—strangely, beautifully—liberating.

This book is for caregivers, families, friends, and those walking through the early stages of memory loss. It is not a clinical guide, but a philosophical and emotional map. It does not promise easy answers, but it offers a new relationship with uncertainty. It's for those ready to flip the script—not to deny the sorrow, but to welcome the joy that still pulses underneath.

Each chapter will offer stories, reflections, and practical ways to shift how we view and live this journey. From redefining love and identity, to crafting rituals that honor connection over cognition, to creating spaces where laughter and play are possible even in decline—this book is your invitation to approach memory loss not just as an end, but as a mysterious, sacred unfolding.

In a society obsessed with productivity, legacy, and personal achievement, Alzheimer's can feel like a cruel dismantling. But in another frame, it can be a call to presence, to surrender, to rediscover the soul beneath the story. As we accompany our loved ones—and ourselves—through this great unwinding, may we do so with open eyes, softened hearts, and deep appreciation.

Let us not only grieve what is lost, but celebrate what is revealed.

Let us enter the grace of forgetting.

Chapter 1: A New Lens on Memory Loss

Reframing Forgetting as a Path to Presence

The diagnosis often comes like a thunderclap. One moment, life is moving forward—maybe slowly, maybe with some stumbles and misplaced keys—but still with continuity. Then, a word is spoken: *Alzheimer's*. Or *dementia*. And in that instant, everything shifts. The future rearranges itself into a horizon of fear. The past starts to tremble with uncertainty. For many, it's the beginning of what feels like a long descent into shadow.

But what if that diagnosis, instead of being a pronouncement of doom, could be a doorway? What if memory loss is not just the erasure of a life, but an opportunity to live it differently, even more fully? What if the unraveling of the mind could offer a kind of revelation—one that is painful, yes, but also holy, profound, and strangely beautiful?

This is the lens we will adopt in this book. It does not ignore the suffering, the practical challenges, or the grief that Alzheimer's brings. But it also does not stop there. Instead, it invites us to look more deeply, to widen our view, and to ask: *What is truly lost in memory loss? And what might be found?*

Letting Go of the "Tragedy-Only" Narrative

Western culture clings to the notion of the autonomous, rational self. From early education to retirement planning, we are conditioned to define ourselves by what we *do*, what we *know*, what we *remember*. When memory begins to fade, so does the scaffolding that props up this identity. It's no wonder that we see Alzheimer's as a tragedy—we believe it strips us of everything that makes us *us*.

But is this the only way to see it?

Let's pause and consider: Is a person without memories less worthy of love? Less capable of experiencing joy? Less deserving of presence?

When we fixate on what is lost, we often miss what remains. And even more tragically, we miss what *is still possible.*

If we can begin to shift from a "tragedy-only" narrative to one that holds both sorrow and beauty, we allow for more authentic, compassionate relationships. We make room for wonder, humor, and even grace.

Memory vs. Presence

Memory is powerful—it shapes our sense of self, informs our choices, connects us to loved ones and milestones. But presence is just as powerful, and often undervalued. The person with Alzheimer's may forget the name of their grandchild, but light up at the sound of their laughter. They may not recall a spouse's birthday, but melt into their embrace. This is not a lack of love—it's love experienced in a different register.

When we shift from memory-based relationships to presence-based ones, we stop asking, *"Do you remember me?"* and start asking, *"Can we share this moment together?"*

This shift, though subtle, changes everything. It lessens the sting of being forgotten. It frees caregivers from the burden of correction. It honors the now as a sacred place of connection.

Unlearning Cultural Fear

Our collective fear of memory loss is not innate—it is taught. In the West, aging is often pathologized. Cognitive decline is treated as something shameful, something to be hidden, managed, or mourned in advance. But in many Indigenous cultures and Eastern spiritual traditions, the aging process is revered, even when cognition shifts.

In some Buddhist teachings, for instance, the concept of "no-self" is foundational. Identity is seen as a flowing, impermanent construct, not a fixed possession. The loss of self, in this light, is not a tragedy—it's a spiritual truth that memory loss simply reveals earlier than expected.

In some African and Native traditions, elders are honored not for what they remember, but for who they *are*—vessels of presence, wisdom, intuition, and being. The idea of someone "losing themselves" would make little sense in a culture that never saw selfhood as static to begin with.

If we allow ourselves to absorb these alternative perspectives, we can begin to unlearn the deep cultural dread around forgetting. We can hold a more spacious understanding of what it means to be human.

The Wisdom of the Moment

When memory fades, a different kind of intelligence often emerges. One rooted in emotion, rhythm, and sensation. A person with dementia might not remember their daughter's name, but might hum along perfectly to a lullaby sung decades ago. They might not understand why everyone is upset, but intuitively offer a hug at just the right moment.

These are not meaningless glitches. They are expressions of emotional presence, body memory, and soul wisdom.

As caregivers and loved ones, we have the opportunity to meet people in this space—not to drag them back to our reality, but to join them in theirs. This requires humility. It requires patience. But it also opens the door to moments of unexpected beauty—moments that do not need to be remembered to be real.

Language, Love, and the Unspoken

As verbal language falters, a new kind of language emerges—one of touch, of tone, of energy. A glance, a smile, a shared silence. These become the new grammar of love.

It's easy to grieve the loss of conversation, but what if we celebrated the rise of connection that doesn't rely on words?

In fact, many people report that their relationships with loved ones deepened as Alzheimer's progressed—not because they talked more, but because they learned to *be* together more. To sit in silence. To hold hands. To cry together. To laugh at nothing. These are not lesser experiences—they are profound.

Choosing to See Differently

We cannot always change what is happening. But we can choose how we see it.

This chapter does not deny the losses that come with dementia. The forgetting of names, the fear of disorientation, the grief of watching a loved one change—all of it is real. But alongside this truth is another one: there is beauty here, too. There is connection. There is laughter. There is liberation.

We can hold both.

To adopt a new lens on memory loss is to reclaim agency in how we relate to it. It is an act of resistance against a culture that only values productivity and preservation. It is a decision to find life in the middle of loss.

This is not a detour around grief. It is a pathway through it—toward presence, toward appreciation, and ultimately, toward peace.

In the next chapter, we will dive deeper into the question of identity. If we are not our memories, then who are we? What remains when memory fades? And can the slow unwinding of identity reveal something more eternal beneath?

Chapter 2: Unwinding Identity – What Are We Without Memory?

Reimagining Selfhood in the Absence of Recall

Who are you?

It's a deceptively simple question. For most of us, the answer comes easily: "I'm Jane. I'm a mother, a teacher. I love jazz, hiking, and blueberry pancakes. I was born in 1971. I have two children. I remember my first kiss, my college graduation, and the day my dad died." In essence, we tell our story—we share facts, preferences, memories. We equate *selfhood* with the narrative we've built over time.

But what happens when that story begins to disappear? When the anchor points are no longer accessible? When names slip, and dates blur, and the mirror reflects a face we no longer recognize?

Who are we, then?

This chapter explores a profound and often overlooked aspect of memory loss: the unwinding of identity. As Alzheimer's or other forms of dementia begin to alter cognition, the tightly woven threads that form our self-concept start to unravel. To the Western mind, this is terrifying—like watching a house collapse in slow motion. But what if it is also a revelation? What if who we *truly* are has little to do with memory?

The Western Self: A Narrative Construction

In Western philosophy and psychology, identity is typically framed as a continuous, coherent narrative. We build our selfhood on memory—our recollections of what we've done, where we've been, and how we've changed. We prize stability in personality, consistency in beliefs, and the ability to explain who we are.

In this framework, memory is not just important—it *is* the self. So it's no surprise that when memory falters, we feel as if the person is slipping away.

But this is only one view.

The Fluid Self in Other Traditions

In contrast, many Indigenous, Eastern, and mystical traditions understand the self very differently.

In **Buddhism**, the concept of *anatta*, or "no-self," teaches that there is no fixed, unchanging core of a person. Instead, identity is seen as a collection of constantly shifting perceptions, feelings, and thoughts. Memory is transient. The idea of a permanent, consistent "I" is an illusion. Letting go of that illusion is not a failure—it is a path to liberation.

In **Hinduism**, the *Atman* (soul) is eternal and unchanging, distinct from the mind and body. The self that forgets is not the *true* self—it is merely the outward shell. Beneath memory and personality lies something deeper and untouchable: divine consciousness.

In **many African and Indigenous cultures**, identity is not primarily individualistic but relational. A person is defined not by personal memories but by their role within the community, the rhythms of nature, and the ancestors who live on through them. When memory fades, this web of belonging still holds.

These perspectives open up a radical question: If we are not the stories we remember, then what are we?

Identity as Presence

A person with Alzheimer's may not recall their wedding day. They may not know their own name. But they may smile when held, cry at a sad song, light up at the sound of birdsong or the touch of a loved one's hand. These moments tell us something essential: the core of who we are is not memory—it is *presence*.

Presence is who we are right now, in this breath. It is the capacity to feel, to connect, to sense beauty, to give and receive love—even when language and recall fall away.

This is not a philosophical trick. It is deeply practical. When we relate to people with memory loss as if they *are still fully themselves*—not because they remember the past, but because they *exist in the present*—we restore dignity and connection.

The Illusion of Permanence

There is a poignant irony in how we perceive memory loss. We act as if it breaks some natural law—that the self is supposed to stay whole and knowable. But in truth, identity is always changing.

The person you were at five is not the person you were at twenty-five, or the one you are now. Every experience, every emotion, every loss or gain reshapes the contours of the self. Alzheimer's just accelerates and intensifies this process. It doesn't introduce instability—it reveals it.

To watch someone you love become "different" as their memory fades is heartbreaking—but also, in some sense, no different than what happens to all of us over time. Memory loss brings into focus what is always true: we are in a constant state of becoming.

A Deeper Kind of Knowing

Caregivers often report moments that feel mysterious, even transcendent. A parent who can't remember their child's name will nonetheless comfort them with instinctive tenderness. A person unable to follow a conversation might suddenly say something poetic or profound. These flashes defy logic—but they hint at a different kind of knowing, one that doesn't rely on memory at all.

We might call it *soul memory*, or *body wisdom*, or *emotional intelligence*. It is the self that lives beneath language and timeline. And it can be just as real, if not more so, than the autobiographical self we're used to clinging to.

For Caregivers: Releasing the Burden of Reinforcement

One of the most painful dynamics for caregivers is the urge to constantly *remind*—to help the person "stay themselves" by anchoring them to their past. "Mom, don't you remember? You were a nurse. You loved classical music. Your brother's name was James." These reminders come from love, but they can be exhausting and sometimes harmful.

Because here's the truth: the person may not *need* to remember in order to *be*.

When we release the idea that we must help them "hold on" to their identity, we open space for a different kind of relationship—one grounded not in who they were, but in who they are right now.

This is not abandonment. It is reverence.

Becoming More Than a Story

In many ways, memory loss invites us all—patient, family, caregiver—to move beyond narrative. We are not our resumes. We are not the sum of our achievements. We are not our trauma, our childhoods, or even our triumphs. Those things shape us, yes, but they do not define us.

When memory is stripped away, what remains is something raw and elemental: breath, sensation, connection, spirit.

This can feel like devastation. But it can also feel like truth.

Identity as Liberation

Paradoxically, losing the story of self can be freeing. The person with dementia is not bound by social roles or shame in the same way. They may say things that are wildly honest, do things they never dared before. They may return to simplicity, to childlike wonder. They are not playing a role—they are simply being.

For many, this is one of the gifts of the journey. Yes, there is pain. Yes, there are moments of confusion and sorrow. But there is also release.

For the person letting go of memory, this unwinding of identity can feel like a loosening of heavy garments. And for those watching, if we can shift our lens, we may see not just deterioration, but transformation.

Reflection Questions

As we close this chapter, consider:

- How much of your identity is based on your memories and roles?

- Who would you be if all of those were taken away?

- Have you ever experienced a moment where your sense of self was quiet or still?

- What qualities would you hope others still see in you, even if you no longer "remember" yourself?

In the next chapter, we'll examine the specific cultural narratives in the West that make memory loss feel like a catastrophe—and how these stories shape not only our fear, but our experience of care. By naming these myths, we begin to loosen their grip and open the door to more life-affirming possibilities.

Chapter 3: Western Myths – Fear, Loss, and the Tragedy Narrative

Why We Suffer More Than We Need To

In the West, few diagnoses strike more fear into the heart than Alzheimer's. For many, the very word conjures images of a loved one staring blankly, unable to recognize their children, lost in a world that seems both alien and cruel. The dominant narrative is one of tragedy, grief, and slow disappearance. Memory loss is not just a medical condition—it's a cultural horror story.

But narratives are not objective truths. They are stories we inherit, absorb, and retell. They are shaped by history, economics, religion, and power. And just as they can limit and harm, they can also be rewritten.

In this chapter, we unpack the dominant Western myths around Alzheimer's and memory loss—myths that shape our understanding of identity, value, and care. We examine how these myths feed unnecessary suffering, and how we can begin to disentangle from them, one by one.

The Myth of the Self as a Fixed Story

Perhaps the most deeply rooted Western myth is the idea that our identity is a fixed, coherent, linear narrative.

In this view, we are the sum of our memories and achievements: the places we've been, the things we've done, the roles we've played. We tell our stories with a beginning, middle, and end. And we expect continuity—that who we are at 70 should somehow be traceable back to who we were at 17.

Alzheimer's shatters this assumption. It disrupts the timeline. Suddenly, the person we love doesn't "follow the script." They don't remember their wedding day or their career. They live in the present moment, or in a different decade entirely.

To a culture obsessed with narrative control, this is terrifying. It's seen as the collapse of the self.

But this fear is based on a myth. Identity has never been truly fixed. Our lives are shaped by impermanence and change. We evolve constantly— through heartbreak, love, illness, growth, and loss. Memory loss simply reveals a truth that has always been there: that selfhood is more fluid than we like to admit.

The Myth of Productivity and Worth

Another powerful myth is that our value as human beings lies in what we can *do*. In a capitalist society, productivity is worshiped. We measure people by their output—their job, their efficiency, their contribution. Retirement is often seen as a slow fade into irrelevance. And dementia? As a final, tragic exit from the economy of usefulness.

This mindset is cruel, especially to the elderly. It implies that once someone can no longer "contribute," they no longer matter. They become a burden, rather than a being with intrinsic worth.

But worth is not conditional. It does not depend on memory, language, or independence. Every person—at every stage of life and cognition—is inherently valuable. A newborn is not "useful," yet we love them fiercely. Why do we not extend that same reverence to an elder who is letting go of memory?

When we strip away the myth of productivity as identity, we can begin to see people as they are—not as what they do or remember, but as sacred beings, worthy of care and connection.

The Myth of Control

Western culture places high value on autonomy, independence, and control. We are taught to plan for the future, manage risk, and stay in charge of our bodies and minds. Dementia is terrifying in part because it feels like a loss of this control. You can't plan your way out of it. You can't "will" your brain to remember.

This myth makes memory loss feel like failure. Not just illness, but *personal failure*. It feeds shame and stigma—for those experiencing the condition and those caring for them.

But in truth, control has always been an illusion. Life is unpredictable. Aging brings change. Illness is part of the human condition. Rather than fighting this truth, we can learn to surrender to it—not in defeat, but in humility. In openness.

Some of the most beautiful moments in dementia care come when people stop trying to force clarity or correctness, and instead meet their loved one where they are—with curiosity, compassion, and presence.

The Myth of the "Empty Shell"

One of the most damaging metaphors in dementia discourse is the idea that the person becomes an "empty shell"—as if the soul has departed while the body lingers.

This dehumanizing image is not only painful, it is false.

People with memory loss still feel, still respond to love and music and beauty. They may not be able to express themselves as before, but that does not mean they are absent. They are still *there*—in different ways, on different frequencies.

17

Seeing someone as "gone" long before their death robs them—and us—of the rich possibility of connection in the present moment.

It also justifies neglect. If the person is already "gone," why bother reaching for them? Why make the effort? This belief leads to abandonment, loneliness, and emotional harm.

To reject the "empty shell" myth is to commit to seeing the whole person, again and again, regardless of what they remember.

The Myth of Dignity as Competence

Dignity, in Western thought, is often linked to independence, rationality, and control. The ability to speak clearly, manage one's affairs, and maintain composure is seen as the hallmark of a dignified life.

So when someone begins to lose words, forget faces, or need assistance with daily care, we assume their dignity is diminished. We talk about "preserving dignity" as if it were a fragile possession slipping away.

But dignity is not lost with memory. It does not vanish with confusion. It lives in how we treat one another—in the respect we offer, the patience we bring, the care we extend.

To truly honor dignity, we must redefine it. Not as the ability to perform, but as the inherent worth of being human.

The Cultural Fear of Death

At its core, much of the fear around Alzheimer's is tangled up with our fear of death. Memory loss is seen as a kind of premature dying—a slow disappearance of the self before the body is ready to let go.

But perhaps this is a misunderstanding.

In many spiritual traditions, death is not the enemy. It is part of the cycle. A transition. A return. Dementia, from this perspective, might be seen not as a loss, but as a form of passage. A spiritual unwinding. A gradual loosening of the ego in preparation for something more mysterious.

This is not to romanticize suffering. But to acknowledge that our terror of forgetting is also a terror of mortality. When we begin to relate to death differently, we may find a gentler way to relate to memory loss as well.

Challenging the Tragedy-Only Narrative

The collective myths described above form the backbone of what we might call the "tragedy-only" narrative. This is the story that says Alzheimer's is nothing but loss. That life after diagnosis is a slow, humiliating fade. That caregivers are martyrs. That joy is no longer possible.

This narrative dominates media, fundraising campaigns, medical discourse, and popular imagination. And while it captures real pain, it leaves out just as much.

It leaves out laughter. Moments of unexpected clarity. Touch, music, rhythm, spirit. It leaves out the ways people with dementia continue to teach us—to slow down, to let go, to live in the now.

It also leaves out transformation. Not just of the person with memory loss, but of everyone around them. Many caregivers speak of becoming more patient, more present, more emotionally attuned. Some even call it holy.

Rewriting the Story

We need new narratives. Not ones that erase suffering, but ones that tell a fuller truth. Stories where memory loss is not the end of meaning, but the beginning of a different kind. Stories where caregivers are not saints or victims, but companions in a sacred unfolding. Stories where presence matters more than memory, and love needs no timeline to endure.

By exposing the myths that shape our fear, we free ourselves to imagine and live new possibilities.

Practices for Shifting the Narrative

1. **Notice Your Language:** Replace terms like "he's gone" with "he's changed." Say "she's in a different place now" rather than "she's lost herself."

2. **Find Role Models:** Seek out books, films, or communities that portray dementia with nuance, humor, and dignity. Normalize seeing beauty and connection in this journey.

3. **Challenge Stereotypes:** When you hear others speak of memory loss as only tragic, gently offer another perspective. Share a meaningful moment or story that defies the trope.

4. **Honor Moments, Not Memories:** Begin to orient around shared presence rather than shared history. Celebrate the now.

In the next chapter, we will explore the liberating potential of letting go. What might Alzheimer's teach us about surrender, simplicity, and spiritual freedom? Can the unraveling of memory become a path—not to despair—but to inner release?

Chapter 4: Liberation Through Letting Go

Releasing the Illusion of Control and Embracing the Sacred Simplicity of Now

---

To most people, the phrase "letting go" in the context of Alzheimer's and memory loss sounds like an admission of defeat. It evokes images of giving up hope, losing grip on reality, or surrendering to a process we fear and hate. In a society that equates holding on with strength, letting go seems like the opposite of love.

But what if we have it backward?

What if letting go is not failure, but freedom? What if release is not abandonment, but an invitation—to simplicity, to presence, to the essence of who we really are beneath the clutter of memory, identity, and control?

In this chapter, we explore the paradox of liberation through loss. We unpack how the unraveling of memory—both for the person experiencing it and those caring for them—can become an unexpected doorway into a lighter, more peaceful way of being.

The Constant Effort of Holding On

From the moment we learn to speak, we begin building stories—about ourselves, our families, our pasts, our ambitions. These stories are stitched together with memory. We learn to perform roles: daughter, father, teacher, artist, leader. These roles come with expectations, responsibilities, and often, emotional armor.

As we age, we continue carrying these layers. For many, it's exhausting. The mind becomes a busy highway of to-do lists, regrets, self-judgment, and anticipation. We define ourselves by our accomplishments and our accumulated identities. To forget, in this context, feels like falling apart.

But underneath that constructed self, there is something else. Something quieter. Something deeper.

Memory loss, for all its grief, begins to peel away the layers. First, the names. Then, the dates. Then the self-protective roles. What remains is not nothingness—but often a startling simplicity.

And within that simplicity, there is space. Space to breathe. To be.

The Gift of Simplicity

Consider this: a person with Alzheimer's may not remember their birthday, but they may delight in the taste of a ripe peach. They may not recall a family vacation, but they may stare for minutes at the flicker of sunlight on the floor. They may not be able to finish a sentence, but they might laugh at the sound of a baby giggling or start humming a familiar melody without prompting.

These are not meaningless scraps. They are moments of unfiltered life. Moments that many of us, in our fully "functioning" minds, rush past every day.

Memory loss can pull us—and those around us—into a new kind of rhythm. Slower. Softer. Present. It can strip away what is unnecessary, leaving behind a kind of sacred minimalism.

It doesn't make the pain go away. But it reveals something else: that much of what we thought we needed to be "whole" was not essential after all.

Caregiving as a Practice of Surrender

Caregivers, too, often speak of this shift. At first, there is resistance: the effort to fix, to correct, to explain, to keep the person tethered to "reality." But over time, many realize that reality is no longer a fixed place. And that the more they try to pull their loved one back, the more suffering they both endure.

The turning point often comes when caregivers stop trying to hold on—and instead *join* their loved one wherever they are.

This surrender is not passive. It is powerful. It means meeting someone with openness rather than expectation. It means letting go of needing to be understood in conventional ways. It means trusting that love does not depend on recognition.

For many caregivers, this moment of letting go—though born from fatigue or heartbreak—becomes the beginning of a new kind of intimacy. A deeper form of love.

One that is not transactional. One that is not dependent on past or future. One that simply *is*.

Letting Go of the Need to Be Right

One of the unexpected gifts of memory loss is that it teaches those around it to loosen their grip on "rightness."

In daily interactions, especially early in the disease, a person might misremember events, confuse people, or invent alternate versions of the truth. The reflexive response is to correct: "No, Mom, it wasn't Dad who took you to the dance—it was Uncle Joe." "You didn't live in Chicago, you lived in Detroit." "That didn't happen. You're remembering it wrong."

But what if "rightness" doesn't matter?

What if the emotional truth of the moment—the joy, the fear, the warmth—is more important than factual accuracy? What if we stop trying to anchor people in our version of reality, and instead float gently with them in theirs?

This kind of letting go is a liberation not only for the person with dementia but for those in relationship with them. It creates space for play, for creativity, for meeting without the pressure of mutual understanding. It allows us to be, instead of always doing or fixing.

Dismantling the Ego, Softening the Self

In many spiritual traditions, the ego is seen as the source of suffering. The ego craves control, certainty, and validation. It wants to be seen, remembered, understood, and appreciated. It panics at the idea of being forgotten or fading away.

Alzheimer's, in this light, becomes a profound ego dismantler.

For the person experiencing it, the loss of self-image and social status can feel like humiliation at first. But eventually, many reach a place of peace—a childlike state where they are no longer performing. They are no longer trying to impress, achieve, or maintain a persona. They simply *are*.

For those caring for them, the ego also softens. There is less room for pride or control. Caregiving demands humility. It asks you to be patient when you are exhausted, to offer love even when it is not returned in the way you expect.

It is brutal at times. But it is also alchemical.

Both parties are slowly reshaped—not by effort, but by the experience of loosening. In the absence of ego, what emerges is not nothingness, but tenderness.

Liberation from Time

In a culture obsessed with schedules, goals, and future planning, dementia offers something countercultural: a life lived outside of time.

People with advanced memory loss often dwell in nonlinear reality. They may shift between past and present, between dream and wakefulness. They may forget that hours have passed, or repeat the same question dozens of times in a minute.

To the rational mind, this is maddening. But to the heart, there is an opportunity here.

If we stop fighting the clock—and instead enter into this timelessness— we may discover a kind of peace. A rhythm less about what comes next and more about what is now.

There is a certain freedom in forgetting the future. In not worrying about what's ahead. In not organizing experience around outcomes. It's a kind of spiritual surrender. A release of the mind's tyranny over being.

This freedom is frightening—but also sacred. In it lies the possibility of true presence.

Letting Go as a Shared Journey

Ultimately, the letting go that happens in Alzheimer's is not one-sided. It is mutual. The person with memory loss lets go of identity, chronology, and control. Their loved ones let go of expectations, roles, and the need to be remembered.

And in this shared surrender, something tender and unexpected can arise: a deeper kind of relationship.

One not based on shared history, but on shared humanity. Not on past meaning, but on present connection.

This doesn't mean pain disappears. Grief still comes. Moments of clarity can bring fresh sorrow. But beneath the pain, there can also be joy. And laughter. And peace.

Not because forgetting is easy—but because letting go is sometimes the most loving thing we can do.

Practices in Letting Go

1. **Sit Without Correcting:** The next time your loved one misremembers something, resist the urge to correct them. Instead, follow the thread. Ask questions. Let their version of reality unfold.

2. **Release the Schedule:** Choose one day a week to let go of time. Follow their rhythm. Don't rush. Don't plan. Just be.

3. **Breathing Meditation:** Practice a simple breathing meditation. Inhale: "Let." Exhale: "Go." Allow yourself to soften. Practice not knowing. Just for a few minutes.

4. **Touchstone Object:** Find a small object that represents release for you—a smooth stone, a feather, a leaf. Keep it nearby to remind yourself of the beauty in surrender.

In Closing

Letting go is often painted as a loss. And it is. But it is also a door. One that opens into unexpected peace, simplicity, and connection.

In the journey through memory loss, we may lose names, places, and narratives. But we may also lose anxiety. Perfectionism. Control. The need to be understood.

In their place, we may find something else: presence. Grace. And a love that needs no memory to endure.

In the next chapter, we will explore how living in the *moment*—rather than clinging to memory—can become the cornerstone of joyful connection. It's not about remembering life; it's about experiencing it, now.

Chapter 5: Moments Over Memory – The Power of the Present

Why Presence, Not the Past, Is the True Gift of Connection

There is a quiet revolution waiting inside every moment we share with someone whose memory is fading. It happens when we stop asking, *"Do you remember?"* and start asking, *"Are you here with me now?"*

For those living with Alzheimer's or other forms of dementia, the present moment can become the only real home. Past and future grow hazy or disappear altogether, while the now pulses with intensity—sometimes disorienting, sometimes magical. What we often call "attention deficit" or "confusion" may, in truth, be a radical form of presence.

As caregivers, family, and friends, we often approach Alzheimer's from the rearview mirror: grieving what's lost, trying to reinforce what was. But the more we try to drag people back into memory, the more we risk missing the sacredness of what's unfolding right in front of us.

This chapter invites us to flip the script completely. Instead of mourning the absence of memory, we begin to celebrate the miracle of the *moment*. We learn to build relationships not on shared pasts, but on shared *now*. And in doing so, we access a kind of joy and connection that does not require recall—only presence.

The Myth That Connection Depends on Memory

The dominant cultural narrative tells us that memory is the glue of relationship. It's how we track love—through anniversaries, inside jokes, shared vacations, and childhood photos. We believe that to be forgotten is to be unloved. That if someone does not remember who we are, the relationship has disappeared.

But this belief does not hold up in practice.

Many caregivers describe moments when their loved one, despite not knowing their name, still *feels* connected. They reach for your hand. They smile when they see you. They hum along to a familiar tune or mirror your body language in unspoken harmony.

These are not accidents. They are forms of presence-based connection.

We can choose to meet people here, in the space of shared now—not requiring recognition or remembrance to validate the relationship.

Presence does not depend on the past. It only requires *this moment.*

Building a New Language of Connection

When verbal memory fades, a different language becomes possible—one built on intuition, rhythm, sensation, and emotion. You begin to communicate with your eyes, your voice tone, your hands, your breath. You share meaning without words. And often, this kind of connection is *more* honest than what came before.

A person may not remember your name. But they remember your energy.

They respond to your frustration with anxiety. They respond to your calm with calm. They may not track what you're saying, but they *feel* how you're saying it.

This awareness invites us into a higher kind of listening. A softer kind of presence. It asks us to slow down, to tune in—not to memory, but to *feeling.*

In this space, even the smallest acts become profound: brushing someone's hair. Swaying together to a favorite song. Sharing a cookie. Making eye contact. These are not lesser moments. They are sacred.

The Magic of Repetition

One of the hardest aspects of dementia for caregivers is repetition. The same question asked ten times in an hour. The same story told on loop. It can wear down even the most loving heart.

But repetition can also be a form of ritual.

In many spiritual traditions, repetition is not a sign of confusion—it's a path to presence. Think of mantra, prayer beads, breathwork. Think of children's games, where repetition is how play is deepened and joy is sustained.

What if we viewed repetitive questions not as glitches, but as invitations? To answer again with grace. To practice patience. To return, again and again, to presence.

This reframing can reduce frustration and increase empathy. It shifts the energy from correction to communion.

Memory Is Not the Only Form of Knowing

In Western culture, memory is privileged above all other ways of knowing. But people with dementia often retain emotional memory long after episodic memory fades.

They may not remember *why* they love a certain person, but they feel good in their presence. They may forget the *context* of a song, but their body remembers how to dance to it. They may not understand your words, but they sense the safety in your tone.

These forms of knowing are just as valid—sometimes more so. They are primal, embodied, and intuitive.

When we acknowledge these deeper forms of intelligence, we begin to trust the moment more. We stop testing and correcting. We start *being with*.

The Now as Enough

As caregivers and family members, we often feel the ache of all the "used to be's." We miss the person our loved one was before: the sharp wit, the long talks, the shared memories. This grief is real. But it does not have to cancel out the now.

Now may be different—but it is still full of possibility.

Now may be quiet, but it is not empty.

A single shared breath, a gentle smile, a touch on the shoulder—these moments *are enough*. They do not require history. They do not depend on who remembers what. They are real. They are holy.

When we begin to trust the now, we free ourselves—and our loved ones— from the impossible task of trying to hold onto what is already gone.

We make space for what *is still here*.

Practices to Anchor in the Present

Here are some gentle ways to lean into presence with your loved one:

1. **Mirror Play**
   Sit face-to-face and slowly mirror each other's movements— hands, head tilt, blinking, breath. This nonverbal mirroring can build connection, especially when words are elusive.

2. **Sensory Rituals**
   Use touch, smell, and sound to ground in the now. Rub scented

lotion on their hands. Play soft music they once loved. Sit together in sunlight. Let the senses lead.

3. **Three-Word Conversations**
   When language fades, try "conversations" with only three-word phrases: "Nice day today." "You look beautiful." "I love you." These simple phrases can be repeated rhythmically, creating calm and connection.

4. **The Pause Practice**
   Instead of rushing into correcting or explaining, take a conscious breath before responding. Ask: What matters right now? What needs to be said—or not said?

5. **Shared Stillness**
   Sit together in silence. Breathe together. Let the silence be enough.

Shifting from Memory-Based to Moment-Based Love

Our cultural love language is deeply tied to memory. We say: "Remember when we...?" "You always loved..." "We used to..."

But moment-based love is different. It does not ask for history. It simply asks for presence.

Try replacing memory-based expressions with present-focused ones:

- Instead of "Do you remember me?" say, "I'm so happy to see you."

- Instead of "You used to love this song," say, "Let's enjoy this song together."

- Instead of "You forgot my name again," say, "I'm here with you."

This shift takes effort. But it changes everything.

Finding Joy in the Present

The present moment is not a consolation prize—it's the heart of all experience.

We laugh in the present. We cry in the present. We fall in love, we grieve, we wonder—in the present.

For someone with memory loss, the present may be *all* they have. But that is not a deficit. That is an invitation.

If we can join them there—not reluctantly, but wholeheartedly—we may find a kind of joy that doesn't need a name or a reason. A joy that simply *is*.

A New Kind of Legacy

When we focus on memory, we think of legacy as what's left behind: photos, journals, awards, family stories.

But when we focus on the moment, legacy becomes something else: the imprint of love. The warmth someone feels in your presence. The sense of being safe, seen, cherished.

You don't have to be remembered to leave a mark.

Sometimes, just being present is the legacy.

In Closing

Memory loss challenges us to redefine what matters in relationship. When we let go of needing to be remembered, we open the door to being truly *received.* When we stop insisting on shared past, we discover the wonder of shared *now.*

In this new light, connection is not lost—it is transformed.

You don't need to remember the moment for it to be real. You only need to *live* it.

In the next chapter, we'll look beyond Western culture to explore how other societies understand aging and memory loss. What can we learn from traditions that honor forgetting not as a loss, but as a return to essence?

Chapter 6: Spiritual Echoes – Cultural Wisdom from Other Traditions

Seeing Forgetting as a Sacred Path, Not a Tragic Ending

In the West, memory loss is often met with panic, pity, and the language of tragedy. We scramble for cures, mourn prematurely, and frame Alzheimer's as an enemy to be conquered. But this view is not universal.

Around the world, across centuries, many cultures have held entirely different relationships with aging, forgetting, and the transformation of the mind. Some view these shifts not as disease but as stages of sacred transition. Others see the waning of memory not as loss, but as a return— to soul, to spirit, to a more intuitive or essential self.

In this chapter, we travel beyond the Western biomedical model. We listen to the spiritual echoes in Indigenous, Eastern, African, and mystical traditions. What emerges is a powerful, liberating reframe: that memory loss, rather than stripping away identity, may reveal a deeper kind of wisdom. A kind of coming home.

Indigenous Perspectives: Elderhood as Transformation

In many Indigenous cultures, elderhood is a revered stage of life. It is not defined by what one remembers, but by the role one plays in the community and the wisdom one carries—wisdom that does not always rely on words.

Among the **Diné (Navajo)** people, for example, age is not equated with decline but with spiritual depth. A person who no longer speaks much, who sits in long stretches of silence, may be understood as entering a phase of listening—to the ancestors, the land, or spirit.

In some **Australian Aboriginal** cultures, dreaming is a central concept: a state where the boundaries of time blur and ancestral knowledge flows freely. Older adults who move between present and dream-like states are not pitied but respected. Their altered perception is not always corrected—it is honored.

In these traditions, forgetting is not always a problem to solve. Sometimes, it's a shift in consciousness—a movement from linear time to sacred time. The person is not "gone." They are *going somewhere else.*

Eastern Philosophy: Losing Self as Gaining Truth

In **Buddhism**, the concept of *anatta*—no fixed self—sits at the heart of spiritual awakening. According to this teaching, the idea of a consistent, separate identity is an illusion. Our thoughts, memories, and even personalities are constantly shifting. Suffering arises when we cling to them as if they were permanent.

Seen through this lens, the process of memory loss is not inherently tragic. It can be a form of letting go of ego, of story, of illusion. It can be a spontaneous entry into a kind of spiritual simplicity—where the past drops away and only being remains.

Some Buddhist teachers describe the late stages of Alzheimer's as akin to a meditative state: the person no longer filters life through conceptual thinking, but lives through sensation, rhythm, and presence. This is not to deny the challenges—but to reframe the condition as holding potential for awakening, not just deterioration.

In **Taoism**, similarly, the path to harmony lies in yielding, not resisting. As memory fades, the person may become more aligned with *wu wei*—the Taoist principle of effortless flow. They are no longer striving or performing. They simply *are.*

African Wisdom Traditions: Personhood as Belonging

In many African cultures, identity is not an individual possession but a communal phenomenon. The phrase **"I am because we are"** (from the Ubuntu philosophy) captures this beautifully. A person exists through relationship, through belonging, through connection to others.

This worldview stands in stark contrast to the Western ideal of selfhood as solitary achievement. In Ubuntu, you are not defined by what you remember, but by how you are held in the hearts of your community.

An elder with memory loss, therefore, is not "losing themselves"— because their self was never entirely theirs to begin with. It lives in the songs, stories, and memories of the tribe. Their value does not diminish. Their dignity does not depend on independence.

They are remembered *into* being.

Sufism and Mystical Christianity: Ecstasy in Unknowing

In mystical traditions, forgetting is often revered—not as decline, but as divine union.

In **Sufi** poetry, the self is seen as something to be forgotten so that one may merge with the Beloved (God). The great Sufi mystic Rumi writes:

"Try to be like the sun: come to the light without memory."

To forget, in this view, is not an error—it is transcendence.

Similarly, in **Christian mysticism**, saints like St. John of the Cross and Meister Eckhart speak of *unknowing* as a spiritual virtue. True wisdom comes not through accumulated knowledge, but through the surrender of it. The mystic does not ascend by remembering more—but by letting go of mental constructs, entering the silence of the soul.

What if dementia, at its most mysterious, echoes this process?

Of course, Alzheimer's is not a chosen spiritual practice. But these teachings remind us: there is precedent for seeing forgetting as sacred. There is space for awe, even in the unraveling.

Music, Touch, and Soul Memory

Across traditions, certain forms of memory are considered deeper than mind.

Music, for instance, often remains accessible long after names and dates have disappeared. Songs heard in childhood can stir recognition and emotion. A drumbeat can animate the body, awaken joy, summon tears.

This has led some to speak of **"soul memory"**—the idea that certain patterns and feelings are stored in the heart, the body, or the spirit.

In **African diasporic religions**, rhythm and dance are used not only to remember ancestors, but to *become* them. Movement carries memory that the tongue forgets.

In **Indigenous ceremonies**, touch is often the language of prayer. Hands on shoulders, the brushing of hair, the sharing of food—all communicate care, memory, and meaning.

These traditions teach us that presence is not limited to cognitive recall. It can be felt. Transmitted. Known without knowing how.

What We Can Learn

Western medicine has its strengths. It offers research, structure, support, and insight into brain function. But it often lacks spiritual imagination. It sees memory loss only as pathology, never as passage.

By listening to other traditions, we can:

- **Expand our definitions of identity**, moving beyond the brain to include the body, community, and spirit.

- **Reframe memory loss as a sacred process**, not just a medical condition.

- **Honor intuitive and non-verbal forms of connection**, such as touch, music, and ritual.

- **Recognize that value and dignity are not dependent on cognition.**

This does not mean romanticizing suffering. It means holding space for *meaning* within it. It means allowing spiritual interpretations to sit alongside scientific ones.

It means asking not just, *"How do we treat this?"* but also, *"What is this teaching us?"*

Creating Rituals of Reverence

Inspired by these traditions, here are some ways to bring spiritual wisdom into daily care:

1. **Create a "sacred space" corner.** A chair by a window, a favorite blanket, fresh flowers, or a photo can signal a place of peace. Return here daily to breathe, connect, and simply *be*.

2. **Use music as prayer.** Find songs from your loved one's childhood, faith, or culture. Sing them together. Hum. Let the rhythm speak.

3. **Honor touch.** A daily hand massage, hair brushing, or gentle hug can become a ritual of love that goes beyond language.

4. **Tell communal stories.** Share memories of your loved one in community. Let others carry the remembering for them. Let memory become collective, not personal.

5. **Sit in silence.** Light a candle. Say nothing. Be present. Know that presence itself is holy.

In Closing

The Western fear of forgetting is not inevitable—it is cultural. And culture can change.

By drawing from the spiritual echoes of other traditions, we begin to unlearn the belief that memory defines the self. We open to the idea that forgetting may be a sacred return: to essence, to presence, to the love that has no need for names.

There is deep wisdom in the world's oldest teachings—wisdom that reminds us: the person we love is not disappearing. They are changing form. And if we can meet them in the space beyond story, we may find that they are still here, shining.

Not in memory, perhaps.

But in spirit.

In the next chapter, we'll bring these insights down to earth. We'll explore what it means to *care* for someone not by trying to correct or fix them—but by connecting with them exactly where they are. This is the art of relational care—not technical care, but *human* care.

Chapter 7: Care as Connection, Not Correction

Meeting People Where They Are, Not Where We Think They Should Be

---

In the early stages of dementia caregiving, many of us operate from a well-intentioned instinct: to *help our loved ones stay oriented*. We want to correct their memory slips, remind them of the facts, ground them in "reality." We say, "No, that's not right," or "You're forgetting again," or "We've already talked about that." We do this with love, with hope, even with desperation. It feels like the right thing.

But here's the truth: correction often leads to frustration, not clarity. It increases anxiety. It causes embarrassment. It can damage trust.

Why? Because the cognitive world we're asking them to return to no longer feels accessible. For the person with Alzheimer's or dementia, time becomes elastic. Memory becomes fragile. What we call "the truth" may feel distant or irrelevant.

When we correct, we push them into a world they no longer understand. But when we connect—we enter theirs.

This chapter is about shifting the caregiving paradigm: from managing behavior to meeting emotion, from correcting facts to cultivating presence. It's about relational care—the kind that honors dignity, fosters connection, and builds bridges not through logic, but through love.

Correction: The False Promise of Control

It's tempting to think that if we could just remind our loved one enough—show them the right pictures, give them the right cues—they would snap back into clarity. And sometimes, in the early stages, reminders *do* help. Structured environments, calendars, gentle prompts—these can offer support.

But over time, correction becomes less effective and more harmful. Here's why:

- **It assumes the person can rejoin our timeline**—when often, they've slipped into another.

- **It centers the caregiver's need for reality**, not the person's need for reassurance.

- **It can make the person feel small, ashamed, or "wrong."**

- **It misses the emotional truth in favor of factual correctness.**

A person who insists they need to "go home" might be speaking less about geography and more about a feeling—safety, familiarity, love. Arguing with them about their address misses the point. But offering comfort, asking what home means, or sitting quietly with them can meet the deeper need.

Connection: The Power of Joining, Not Redirecting

Connection asks a different question: *What is this person feeling, and how can I meet them there?*

Instead of pulling them into our world, we step into theirs.

This doesn't mean pretending. It means honoring the *reality of the moment*, as it exists in their experience.

Here are examples of shifting from correction to connection:

- **Instead of:** "Mom, Grandma died ten years ago. You forgot again."
  Try: "You miss her a lot, don't you? Tell me about her."

- **Instead of:** "We already had lunch! Don't you remember?"
  Try: "You're hungry? Let's get a snack."

- **Instead of:** "That's not your baby—that's a doll."
  Try: "She's beautiful. Would you like to hold her?"

Each of these moments becomes a bridge. You're not reinforcing facts—you're reinforcing *connection*.

The Emotional Landscape of Memory Loss

People with dementia may forget *what* happened, but they often remember *how they felt*.

If an interaction made them feel safe, valued, or loved, that emotional imprint stays. If it made them feel criticized, belittled, or confused—that, too, remains.

Emotional memory outlasts cognitive memory.

This is why caregiving rooted in correction can unintentionally sow trauma. A person may not remember the conversation, but their body may hold onto the tension, the fear, the shame.

Conversely, care grounded in kindness and connection can create a residual sense of safety—even when specifics are forgotten.

Relational Care vs. Clinical Care

Clinical care focuses on tasks: hygiene, medication, nutrition, safety. These are vital, of course. But relational care goes deeper. It asks:

- How do I create emotional safety?

- How do I honor the person's dignity?

- How can we experience joy together?

- How do I *be with* them, not just *do for* them?

This shift doesn't require more time. It requires more attention. It's not about doing *more*, but doing things *with intention*.

A bath becomes a moment of tenderness.
Brushing hair becomes an act of reverence.
Mealtime becomes a ritual of togetherness.

The "Yes, And" Approach: Borrowed from Improv

The principles of **improvisational theater** offer powerful lessons for dementia care. In improv, actors are trained to use the phrase *"Yes, and…"* to accept and build upon whatever their scene partner offers.

In caregiving, this means:

- Accepting what your loved one says as real *for them*

- Building on it rather than denying or correcting

- Creating shared moments of play, story, or affection

For example:

- If your father thinks he's back in the army barracks, you might say, "Yes, and I bet the coffee was terrible!"

- If your mother insists she needs to catch a train, you might say, "Yes, and while we wait, let's have some tea."

This doesn't mean lying—it means respecting their perception. It's a dance, not a deception.

When Correction *Is* Necessary

There are moments when correction is appropriate—especially for safety. If a person believes they can drive, or is at risk of harm, redirection may be needed.

But even then, we can do it gently.

- **Instead of:** "You can't drive! You'd crash the car!"
  Try: "The car's in the shop right now. Let's take a walk together."

Redirection works best when it *honors emotion* while offering an alternative.

Use distraction not as manipulation, but as a compassionate pivot.

Honoring Dignity Through Connection

The core principle is simple: *The person is not the problem.* The disease is. And our job is not to pull them back into our world—but to meet them in theirs, without judgment or shame.

When we stop correcting, we give the person freedom to be exactly where they are.

We affirm their reality.

We say, "You matter—not because you remember me, but because you are *you*, right now, in this moment."

Practices for Connection-Based Care

1. **Start with Feeling, Not Fact**
   When responding to confusion or distress, first reflect emotion. "That sounds scary." "You seem upset." "You're excited!"

2. **Use Gentle Curiosity**
   Instead of correcting, ask open-ended questions. "Tell me more about that." "What do you see?" "How does that feel?"

3. **Slow Your Tempo**
   Speak more slowly. Use fewer words. Pause. Wait. Let the space fill naturally.

4. **Celebrate Small Joys**
   Did they smile at a bird outside? Laugh at a silly sound? These are wins. Mark them. Repeat them.

5. **Create Repetition Rituals**
   Lean into favorite stories or questions. Make them part of the rhythm, not a mistake to fix.

6. **Reflect, Don't React**
   When frustrated, ask yourself: "Am I trying to correct… or connect?" Recenter your intention.

In Closing

Relational care is not about fixing—it's about *being with*. It requires patience, empathy, and a willingness to let go of the need to be right.

When we prioritize connection over correction, we give our loved ones something more precious than facts: we give them safety, respect, and belonging.

We affirm that they are not broken. They are human.

Still reachable.

Still worthy.

Still here.

In the next chapter, we'll explore how love can evolve beyond words and roles—how presence, intuition, and emotional attunement can allow relationships to deepen, even as language and memory begin to fade.

Chapter 8: Relearning Love – Emotional Presence Beyond Cognition

Loving Without Labels, Roles, or Words

What does it mean to love someone who no longer remembers you?

This question haunts many families living through the stages of Alzheimer's and dementia. The pain of being forgotten by a spouse, a parent, or a dear friend cuts deep. It's not just memory that fades—it feels like love itself is slipping away.

But love is more than memory.

And this chapter is an invitation to reimagine what love can be when we move beyond cognition—beyond language, beyond roles, beyond expectation. It's about discovering a deeper, more intuitive form of connection that does not depend on recognition, but on *presence*.

Love, it turns out, is not stored in the brain alone. It lives in the body, in the breath, in the spaces between words. And even when memory fails, love can remain—transformed, but no less real.

The Grief of Being Forgotten

Before we explore the possibilities, we must name the grief.

When someone you love forgets your name, it hurts. When they confuse you with someone else, or don't recognize you at all, it can feel like a kind of death—a loss of mutual history, of intimacy, of self.

There's no pretending this isn't hard.

Caregivers often describe a "living grief"—mourning someone who is still alive. And in that mourning, questions arise: *Am I still a daughter if she no longer remembers giving birth to me? Am I still a husband if he doesn't know we're married? Is there still love if there's no recognition?*

The answer is: yes.

But it may not look the way we're used to. It may require letting go of the way we once received love—and learning how to feel it in new, unfamiliar forms.

The Body Remembers What the Mind Forgets

While cognitive memory may deteriorate, emotional memory often persists.

A person with dementia might forget your name but still light up when they see your face. They might not be able to articulate why they feel safe with you—but their body knows. They lean in. They smile. They relax.

This is because the *limbic system*—the emotional brain—remains active long after other regions decline. Touch, tone, facial expression, and rhythm continue to communicate long after language fades.

This means that love is not erased by memory loss—it simply shifts channels.

Instead of verbal reassurances, there is eye contact.

Instead of shared stories, there is shared presence.

Instead of "I love you," there is a held hand, a warm blanket, a gentle smile.

Moving from Role-Based Love to Essence-Based Love

In our relationships, we often love through *roles*: mother, son, spouse, friend. These roles carry expectations—of mutual recognition, shared history, verbal affirmation.

When memory loss blurs these roles, we are invited into something deeper: *essence-based love.*

This is love that is not about who we are *to* each other, but who we are *with* each other.

It's less about history, and more about *presence*.

It's less about what we say, and more about what we *feel*.

It's the kind of love that does not need explanation. It just *is*.

The Intuitive Language of Love

As cognition changes, new forms of communication emerge—forms that rely not on intellect but on intuition.

Some examples:

- **Tone of voice.** A calm, soothing voice can express more love than words.

- **Facial expression.** A warm smile, raised eyebrows, or soft eyes can create deep connection.

- **Touch.** A light hand on the shoulder, a hug, a held hand can communicate safety and affection.

- **Music.** Singing or humming a familiar tune can awaken emotion and spark joy.

- **Shared rhythm.** Rocking in chairs together, breathing in sync, or dancing slowly can create attunement beyond words.

These gestures are not secondary. They are the *primary* language of love when cognition declines.

They allow the relationship to continue—even deepen—without memory or conversation.

Reframing Love from Memory to Presence

We often think love lives in the past: in the anniversaries, the shared jokes, the inside references. But love also lives right here, in this breath.

Here are ways to shift from memory-based love to presence-based love:

- **Instead of:** "Remember when we used to…"
  Try: "This moment with you feels good."

- **Instead of:** "Don't you know who I am?"
  Try: "I love being here with you."

- **Instead of:** "You forgot me again."
  Try: "I'm here, and I'm staying with you."

These reframes take courage. They ask us to release the desire to be known in a certain way—and to accept being loved in a new one.

Love as Practice, Not Proof

One of the hardest shifts in dementia caregiving is learning to give love *without needing proof of return*.

This doesn't mean becoming a martyr. It doesn't mean ignoring your own need for recognition or appreciation. But it does mean finding ways to root love in *action*, not just affirmation.

Love becomes a practice:

- Sitting together without needing conversation.

- Offering care without expecting thanks.

- Listening for the emotion beneath the confusion.

- Being willing to show up, again and again, even when the person no longer knows your name.

In this way, love becomes less about exchange and more about presence. Less about being remembered, and more about being real.

Mutual Transformation

While it may seem that only the person with dementia is changing, caregivers often undergo profound transformation as well.

They speak of becoming more patient. More attuned. More emotionally sensitive. More spiritually open.

They learn to slow down. To savor small moments. To let go of roles and outcomes.

In relearning love, they are also *being* relearned—shaped into more present, more compassionate versions of themselves.

Love becomes not just something they *give*—but something they *become*.

When Words Return

Sometimes, in the fog of late-stage dementia, a moment of clarity emerges. A person who hasn't spoken for days suddenly says, "I love you." Or they call you by name. Or they sing a song you used to sing together.

These moments are gifts.

But they are not *more* real than the silences that came before. They are part of the tapestry, not its only bright thread.

Even when love is not spoken, it is still present.

Even when recognition fades, relationship endures.

Practices for Deepening Emotional Presence

1. **Eye-to-Eye Time**
   Sit face-to-face for five minutes. Don't talk. Just breathe. Notice what changes in your body and theirs.

2. **Touch with Intention**
   Massage their hands with lotion. Let the touch be slow, respectful, and tender.

3. **Tone Mapping**
   Notice how your tone of voice affects their response. Try speaking softly, with warmth and ease.

4. **Daily Presence Ritual**
   Choose a small, daily ritual—lighting a candle, sharing a piece of fruit, singing a song—that becomes your moment of connection.

5. **Loving Without Being Known**
   Reflect on this: *Can I still love if I am not remembered?* Journal your response. Let it evolve over time.

In Closing

Alzheimer's asks us to let go of many things. But it also asks us to *return*—to presence, to simplicity, to love that does not require language.

It invites us to love in ways we never expected: intuitively, emotionally, non-verbally. It invites us to be known not by name, but by energy. Not by role, but by feeling. Not by memory, but by *presence*.

This is not lesser love.

It is deeper.

It is real.

It is what remains when everything else falls away.

In the next chapter, we will explore how humor and lightness can become essential tools in navigating the unknown. Even amid confusion and sorrow, there is room for joy—and laughter may be one of the most healing responses of all.

Chapter 9: Laughter in the Fog – Finding Humor in the Unknown

When Confusion Gives Way to Connection Through Joy

Amid the long, unpredictable terrain of memory loss, it might feel inappropriate—or even offensive—to laugh. After all, dementia is serious. Painful. Exhausting. There is confusion. Loss. Grief. How could humor possibly belong here?

And yet, again and again, caregivers and loved ones report moments of laughter. Big belly laughs. Surprising bursts of silliness. Accidental jokes that become daily rituals. These moments do not erase the suffering—but they lighten it. They make space for *humanity* in a process that can otherwise feel dehumanizing.

In this chapter, we explore the healing, connecting, and even *sacred* power of humor in the dementia journey. We'll learn to recognize humor not as denial, but as resilience. Not as disrespect, but as intimacy. And we'll explore how laughter—far from being a distraction—can be a bridge across the fog.

The Gift of Unscripted Living

One of the defining features of dementia is its unpredictability. Conversations don't go the way you expect. Timelines don't hold. Identities are fluid. Reality shifts.

This can be stressful—but it also creates a kind of spontaneous theater. The usual rules of logic and social decorum don't apply. And when we stop resisting this, we start to see the possibility for *play*.

Caregivers sometimes joke that "you never know what version of the story you'll get today." Or that "Dad's invented a new language." These moments, when held with love and curiosity, can bring a lightness that doesn't belittle, but actually *honors* the person's changing mind.

Humor, in this space, becomes less about laughing *at* and more about laughing *with*—together, in the absurd beauty of the moment.

The Neuroscience of Laughter and Memory

Laughter isn't just emotionally healing—it's neurologically beneficial.

Even in the later stages of dementia, the brain's ability to process and respond to humor often remains intact. Studies have shown that:

- **Laughter reduces stress hormones** like cortisol.
- **It increases endorphins**, enhancing mood and emotional bonding.
- **It supports cardiovascular health**, which indirectly benefits brain function.
- **Shared laughter builds connection**, even without words or memory.

In short: humor is not superficial. It is physiological. Emotional. Spiritual. It grounds us in the body and the moment—exactly where people with memory loss already live.

Moments of Unintended Comedy

Anyone who has cared for someone with dementia knows the daily moments that are both confusing and hilarious.

Like the woman who wrapped a banana in a napkin and tucked it in her purse like a newborn. Or the man who insisted his son was the neighbor's plumber, then shared heartfelt gratitude for "fixing the sink" after a haircut.

Or the father who referred to his daughter as "the nice lady who brings the cookies" and declared her "better than the last daughter."

These moments are not cruel. They are surreal, yes—but also strangely profound. They reveal a world untethered from ego or correctness. A world where play can happen *because* reality is fluid.

Using Humor as a Bridge

Caregivers often feel trapped between two modes: serious medical management and deep emotional sorrow. Humor becomes the third way—the human way.

Here's how humor can support connection:

- **Defuses tension.** When repeated questions or outbursts arise, a humorous twist can prevent escalation.

- **Creates mutual joy.** Laughing together reminds both people they are still in relationship.

- **Reframes "mistakes."** A forgotten word becomes an invented one. A backward shirt becomes a fashion statement.

- **Signals love and presence.** Laughter is contagious and relational—it reminds the person that you're *with* them, not just caring *for* them.

Importantly, humor works best when it is *inclusive*, never mocking. It should always be a shared language, not a tool of separation.

The Role of Playfulness in Identity

As cognition shifts, traditional markers of personality may fade. But playfulness often remains.

A person who once told jokes might still delight in wordplay. Someone who loved dancing may begin to wiggle to music in a new, exaggerated way. The essence of their humor remains, even as the delivery changes.

Playfulness is a form of identity beyond memory. When we nurture it, we affirm that the person is still *themselves*—still expressive, still creative, still alive.

It's not about "bringing back" the old personality. It's about *meeting the spark that's still there*, in whatever form it now takes.

Caregiver Humor: Coping Without Guilt

Sometimes, caregivers find themselves laughing *after* the moment—at the absurdity, the awkwardness, the emotional whiplash.

And then they feel guilty.

But here's the truth: **you're allowed to laugh.** It doesn't mean you love them less. It doesn't mean you don't take this seriously. It means you're surviving.

Humor is one of the most ancient forms of resilience. It allows us to breathe, to release, to recover. To feel human in the face of what feels inhuman.

And it's not just for you—it's for the relationship. When caregivers allow themselves to lighten up, even briefly, they become more present, more responsive, and more emotionally sustainable over time.

Making Room for Laughter

Here are a few ways to invite humor and play into daily care:

1. **Yes, And... Play**
   Follow their story—no matter how bizarre—with agreement and amplification. If they say they saw a dinosaur outside, say, "I hope it doesn't eat the roses!"

2. **Create Silly Rituals**
   Make a goofy face every time you serve toast. Invent nicknames for each other. Make up a "secret handshake."

3. **Embrace Role Play**
   If they think they're hosting a dinner party or running a hotel, join them in the role. Be the guest. Be the chef.

4. **Let Go of Correction**
   When something "wrong" happens—milk in the cereal bowl before the cereal, shoes on the wrong feet—don't fix it right away. Smile. Laugh. Let it be what it is.

5. **Celebrate Absurdity**
   When things get ridiculous (and they will), name it gently. "Well, this is a very *creative* way to put on pants!" "We've invented a new language today!"

Laughing Together Is Loving Together

One caregiver shared:

"Mom thought I was her mother again. She kept calling me 'mama' and asking for cookies. At first, I was heartbroken. Then I just went with it. I baked cookies. She beamed. I told her she was the best daughter ever. We laughed until we cried. It was the best afternoon we'd had in years."

That's what humor can do.

It doesn't fix anything. But it *frees* something.

It says: we're still here.

We're still *us*.

We can still find joy—even in the fog.

In Closing

Laughter is not a luxury. It's a form of light. A way to remember that we are more than our diagnoses, more than our roles, more than our losses.

It reconnects us to something ancient and essential: play.

To laugh with someone who is forgetting is not to make light of their experience—it is to *meet them in it* with grace.

So let us give ourselves permission to be silly. To smile at the unexpected. To dance when we don't know the steps. To hold joy alongside sorrow.

The fog of memory may settle, but joy is a lamp we can carry through it.

In the next chapter, we will dive deeper into surrender—not as giving up, but as giving *in* to what is. We'll explore how acceptance, when practiced fully, becomes a profound act of love, trust, and inner freedom.

Chapter 10: The Art of Surrender – Lessons in Acceptance

Letting Go Not as Defeat, But as Devotion

There is a point on the journey through dementia where every effort to restore what was—to maintain routines, reinforce facts, preserve identity—begins to fray. You may find yourself exhausted, explaining something for the tenth time, correcting again and again, and feeling as though you're slipping under the weight of it all.

And then, maybe one day, you stop.

You stop insisting they remember.
You stop forcing the conversation to make sense.
You stop grieving the person they were in every moment of their forgetting.

And in that quiet moment, you enter something else entirely: **surrender.**

In our culture, surrender often carries negative connotations—giving up, giving in, admitting defeat. But in spiritual, emotional, and relational terms, surrender is something much more powerful. It is the conscious choice to release resistance. To stop fighting what *is*. To meet reality with open hands and a soft heart.

This chapter explores surrender not as passivity, but as a profound, loving, and transformative act of care. We'll look at what it means to surrender expectations, roles, and control—and how, in doing so, we open to grace, intimacy, and inner freedom.

Resistance and Its Weight

When memory loss begins to affect a loved one, most caregivers first respond with action. We research. We create systems. We monitor. We correct. We try to *fix* the forgetting.

This is natural—it's how we're conditioned. We live in a world that values control, mastery, and prevention. So we resist. We say:

- "This can't be happening."

- "We need to get her back to how she was."

- "He needs to try harder to remember."

But resistance comes at a cost. It creates tension, conflict, disappointment. It builds a wall between you and the person you're trying so hard to hold onto.

The deeper truth is that **resistance isn't love—it's fear**. And when fear is in charge, connection suffers.

Surrender, on the other hand, begins with this simple truth: *I cannot change what is. But I can choose how I meet it.*

The Power of Radical Acceptance

Radical acceptance is the practice of allowing reality to be exactly as it is—without judgment, denial, or demand. It doesn't mean we like what's happening. It doesn't mean we give up caring. It means we stop insisting that reality match our preferences.

In dementia care, radical acceptance might sound like:

- "This is who she is today."

- "He doesn't remember—but he's still here."

- "We're in a new season of life, and I will meet it with grace."

Accepting that your loved one may not return to who they were is not cruel—it is kind. It allows you to meet them where they *are*, not where you *wish* they were.

And in that meeting, love becomes less about memory and more about presence.

Surrendering Roles and Identities

One of the greatest challenges in dementia caregiving is the shift in roles. A husband becomes a nurse. A daughter becomes a mother. A friend becomes a guardian. These role reversals can feel confusing, even unnatural.

We mourn the loss of shared conversations, reciprocal care, equal partnership.

But what if these changes are not an erasure of love—but an evolution of it?

When we surrender the *form* of the relationship, we make room for its *essence* to shine through. We learn that love doesn't depend on symmetry or tradition—it depends on presence, patience, and mutual humanity.

Yes, the person may forget your name. But if they hold your hand in trust, you are still connected.

Yes, the old conversations may be gone. But if you sit together in silence, the bond endures.

Surrendering old roles doesn't weaken love. It clarifies it.

The Courage of Letting Go

Surrender is not easy. It's not something we do once and move on. It's a practice. A return.

Every time you stop correcting.
Every time you stop forcing a memory.
Every time you breathe instead of bracing.

You surrender again.

This takes courage. It requires that we let go of who we thought we were—protector, fixer, hero—and simply *be* with the person we love. It asks us to exchange certainty for trust.

And it invites us into deeper emotional truths: that love is strongest when it stops trying to control.

Surrendering the Need for Meaning

We want this journey to mean something. We want to understand it. To frame it. To give it language.

But dementia often resists narrative. It doesn't follow arcs. It doesn't reward efforts with closure.

This too must be surrendered.

Instead of asking, "What does this mean?" try asking, "What does this moment ask of me?"

Instead of "Why is this happening?" try "How can I bring love to this?"

Meaning, in dementia care, is not always retrospective. It is not always intellectual. It is often *embodied*—felt in the quiet acts of care, in the repetition of rituals, in the moments of laughter or tears.

Meaning doesn't have to be found. It can be made—right here, in the surrender.

When Surrender Feels Like Loss

There will be days when surrender feels like giving up. Days when acceptance tastes like defeat. That's normal. That's human.

It helps to remember that surrender is not about *resignation*—it's about *alignment*. Aligning your expectations with reality. Aligning your heart with what's possible now.

Even on hard days, you can still surrender without collapsing. You can say:

- "Today is difficult, and I accept that."

- "I'm tired, and I forgive myself for that."

- "I love you, even when I don't know how."

This is emotional maturity. And it grows stronger with practice.

Practical Ways to Cultivate Surrender

1. **The Breath Pause**
   Before responding to a moment of confusion, take a breath. One deep inhale. One slow exhale. Say silently, *"This is where we are."*

2. **Release the Script**
   Let go of how things "should" go. If a conversation veers off track, follow it. If the day falls apart, meet it anyway.

3. **Create a Surrender Mantra**
   Choose a phrase to return to when things feel overwhelming:

- o "Let it be."

- o "I meet you here."

- o "We are both doing our best."

4. **Body Scan for Tension**
   Notice where in your body you're holding on—jaw, shoulders, stomach. Soften there. Breathe. Let go physically to let go emotionally.

5. **Name the Moment**
   "I surrender the need to be understood."
   "I surrender the need for control."
   "I surrender the need for the past."

The Sacredness of Softening

To surrender in love is not to fall apart—it is to soften.

It is to say, "I am no longer fighting the current—I am floating with it."

It is not weakness. It is the deepest kind of strength.

Because in surrender, you stop needing the person to be who they were. You allow them to be who they are. And you allow *yourself* to be changed, too.

This is where the alchemy of caregiving lives—not in control, but in surrender. Not in memory, but in presence.

In Closing

The art of surrender is the art of loving without condition.

It is choosing to show up, again and again, even when the story no longer makes sense. Even when the words are gone. Even when the goodbye has stretched into months or years.

It is trust.

It is presence.

It is peace.

And, perhaps, it is the deepest form of love we ever learn.

In the next chapter, we'll turn our focus outward—to the broader circle of loved ones. How can family and friends remain connected and engaged when they feel uncertain or helpless? What new roles and rituals can emerge to support not just the person with dementia, but everyone in their orbit?

Chapter 11: Redefining the Role of Family and Friends

Creating New Ways to Stay Connected, Involved, and Meaningful

One of the most painful and confusing questions for extended family and close friends in the context of memory loss is this: **"What is my role now?"**

When a loved one no longer remembers your name or forgets your relationship entirely, it's easy to assume you've been "erased." For many, this perceived disappearance leads to quiet withdrawal. Friends stop visiting. Siblings fade into the background. Grandchildren feel awkward or unsure. Even close family members may limit contact, uncertain how to stay involved or afraid they'll only "make things worse."

But while roles inevitably shift with dementia, they don't vanish—they evolve. And when we allow ourselves to grieve the loss of familiar roles while also embracing new ones, a different kind of intimacy becomes possible.

This chapter is a loving call to **re-engage**—not in the way things used to be, but in the way things *can* be now. We'll explore how families and friends can re-enter the picture with purpose, creativity, and presence, offering vital support not just to the person with memory loss, but to the entire caregiving ecosystem.

The Myth of "I Don't Matter Anymore"

Let's begin by dismantling a heartbreaking myth:

"If they don't remember me, there's no point in being there."

This belief is understandable—but false.

Memory is not the only measure of relationship. As we explored in earlier chapters, people with dementia often retain emotional memory, sensory recognition, and body-based associations long after cognitive recall fades.

Your presence *still matters.*
Your energy *still registers.*
Your voice, your touch, your way of being *still connects.*

Even if the person cannot name who you are, they can often feel who you are.

Reframing the Role of Family

Instead of asking, "How can I get them to remember who I used to be?" try asking,

"Who can I be for them now?"

That shift changes everything.

Here are a few evolving roles that family members can embrace:

1. The Presence Companion

You don't need to talk or entertain. Just be there. Sit together. Hold hands. Share a snack. Read aloud. You become a calm, grounding presence in their sensory world.

2. The Joy Bringer

Bring music, stories, pictures, scents, or items that spark happiness. You don't need a script—just bring lightness. Play their favorite childhood tune. Dance together. Tell them they are beautiful.

3. The Ritual Keeper

Create or maintain simple rituals: brushing their hair every Sunday, folding napkins together at lunch, watering plants together. These repeated actions build emotional continuity, even without memory.

4. The Memory Holder

Even if they can't remember their stories, *you can*. Share old photos and stories aloud—not to test them, but to let their history breathe. "Here's the photo from your wedding day. You looked so happy."

5. The Caregiver's Ally

Support the primary caregiver. Offer to sit with your loved one so the caregiver can rest. Bring a meal. Ask how *they* are doing. Emotional and logistical support for caregivers ripples into better care for all.

Friends: Your Role Still Matters

Many friends vanish during the dementia journey—not out of cruelty, but out of fear. They don't know what to say. They worry they'll be awkward. They think the person "won't even notice" they're gone.

But friendship isn't just about shared history—it's about *continued presence*.

Here's how friends can stay involved meaningfully:

- **Show up, even if it's short.** A 10-minute visit matters. A phone call, even if one-sided, matters.

- **Bring sensory joy.** Flowers. Music. A familiar scent. A pet. These offerings create pleasure and recognition beyond words.

- **Don't test memory.** Avoid, "Do you remember me?" Instead, say, "I'm so glad to see you." Affirm the present.

- **Reflect feeling, not facts.** "You look so relaxed today." "You make me smile." Let your tone and presence do the talking.

The Courage to Stay

It takes courage to remain in relationship with someone whose cognition is changing. It's vulnerable. It can be uncomfortable. It might hurt to feel forgotten or dismissed.

But it is *infinitely braver* to stay than to disappear.

Staying doesn't mean showing up perfectly. It means showing up *authentically*.

Bring your awkwardness. Bring your broken heart. Bring your nervous laugh.

Just bring *you*.

Reconnecting Across Generations

Children and grandchildren often feel unsure around a loved one with memory loss. They don't know what's appropriate. They don't want to say the wrong thing. So they often hang back, unsure of their place.

But children are *naturally good at being present*. They don't cling to history or expectations. They are playful, curious, and open—exactly the qualities that create connection.

Here are ways to involve younger family members meaningfully:

- **Arts & Crafts Together:** Simple activities like finger painting, Play-Doh, or coloring can become shared, calming experiences.

- **Read Together:** Children's books, picture books, or rhythmic poetry can bridge communication gaps.

- **Music & Movement:** Dance parties, sing-alongs, and rhythmic clapping games bring mutual joy.

- **Story Time:** Let kids tell their own stories to their loved one. It doesn't matter if they're understood—it's about the *exchange*.

Let children know:

- It's okay if Grandma repeats herself.

- It's okay if Grandpa doesn't remember your name.

- Just being with them is enough.

Navigating Conflict Within Families

The stress of caregiving can fracture even the most loving families. Siblings may disagree about care. Some may pull away. Others may criticize from afar.

This too is part of the journey.

Surrendering to the *new roles* means letting go of who we think others should be—and focusing on who we *can* be in this moment.

Try this:

- **Release resentment.** If a family member is absent, focus on how *you* want to show up—not on controlling others.

- **Invite, don't shame.** Instead of, "You never visit," try, "Would you like to come sit with Dad while I run an errand?"

- **Distribute micro-roles.** One person can make calls. Another can send a weekly photo. Not everyone can do the same kind of caregiving—but almost everyone can *do something*.

Creative Ways to Stay Connected at a Distance

Even if you live far away or can't visit regularly, you can still be an active part of your loved one's world:

- **Send recorded voice messages or videos.** Hearing your voice can spark joy even if they don't fully comprehend the words.

- **Mail tactile gifts.** Soft scarves, textured cards, or scented sachets offer sensory pleasure.

- **Set up a scheduled call or virtual visit.** Even five minutes of connection, regularly, creates rhythm.

- **Support the caregiver.** Send food, gift cards, or letters. Ask them what they need—not just how the person with dementia is doing.

Honoring the Role of Witness

Sometimes, the greatest role a family member or friend can play is that of *witness*. You may not be able to fix or change anything. But your presence affirms:
"You are not alone."

To witness is to say:
"I see you."
"I remember you."
"I love you now, as you are."

This witnessing may feel quiet—but it is *holy work*.

It turns relationship into reverence.

In Closing

As roles shift and stories dissolve, love does not vanish—it *transforms*. Family and friends may no longer be recognized in the traditional way, but they can become anchors of safety, joy, ritual, and presence.

You do not need to be remembered to be *felt*.
You do not need to be perfect to be *needed*.
You do not need to return to the past to make a difference *now*.

In the evolving landscape of dementia, your role is not to be who you were—but to become who your loved one needs you to be, *today*.

That is love in action.

In the next chapter, we will explore the power of rituals and small, joyful traditions. How can we intentionally craft rhythms of connection that bring meaning and beauty into daily life, even when memory fades?

Chapter 12: Rituals of Joy – Building Meaningful New Traditions

Creating Rhythms of Connection When Memory Fades

In a world where so much is being forgotten, rituals help us remember what matters.

Rituals anchor us. They hold space for connection, presence, and meaning—especially when linear memory no longer can. Whether they are grand traditions or simple repeated gestures, rituals offer a sense of familiarity and comfort that transcends time and words.

When someone is living with Alzheimer's or another form of dementia, the old routines may fall away. Holidays become confusing. Birthdays are missed. Family customs may no longer make sense. And this can feel like a loss of identity—not just for the person with memory loss, but for everyone around them.

But here lies a powerful truth: **we can create new rituals.**

We can adapt old ones, simplify others, and invent entirely new practices that center around presence, joy, and sensory connection. These rituals don't rely on memory—they rely on feeling. They don't depend on recognition—they depend on rhythm. They aren't about holding onto the past. They're about *meeting the moment, again and again, with love.*

This chapter is an invitation to become ritual-makers—not just caregivers. You'll learn how to craft meaningful, joyful, and emotionally resonant traditions that sustain connection through every stage of the journey.

Why Rituals Matter in the Context of Memory Loss

Rituals are not just cultural habits—they are emotional containers. They give form to feelings. They help people feel safe, included, and grounded.

For people living with dementia, rituals offer:

- **Predictability:** In a world of cognitive confusion, repetition offers reassurance.

- **Sensory engagement:** Rituals often include smells, textures, sounds, or movements that stimulate embodied memory.

- **Emotional safety:** Repetition without pressure allows connection without the stress of performance or memory.

- **Opportunity for joy:** Rituals can create moments of shared play, peace, and intimacy.

For caregivers and families, rituals are touchstones. They remind us: *even when everything is changing, this moment still belongs to us.*

The Shift from Memory-Based Traditions to Experience-Based Rituals

In the early stages of dementia, familiar traditions may still be meaningful. But over time, detailed customs or complex holiday gatherings can become overwhelming or even distressing.

The key is to shift focus:

- **From history to presence**

- **From formality to feeling**

- **From tradition to intention**

For example:

- Instead of hosting a big holiday meal with extended family, you might bake one familiar pie with your loved one and listen to seasonal music together.

- Instead of decorating a full Christmas tree, you might hang a single ornament each morning for twelve days.

- Instead of retelling a shared family story, you might look through one photo and share how it makes *you* feel in the moment.

The goal is not to recreate the past—but to create *meaning now*.

Elements of a Good Ritual

The most effective rituals in the context of dementia share a few common traits:

1. **Simplicity:** They are easy to do without complex steps or explanations.

2. **Repetition:** They happen regularly, reinforcing emotional recognition even when cognitive memory is absent.

3. **Sensory-Based:** They engage the senses—touch, smell, taste, sound, or sight.

4. **Emotionally Resonant:** They evoke feelings of joy, safety, or calm.

5. **Flexible:** They can be adapted on the fly and don't depend on verbal communication.

Let's look at some examples.

Daily Rituals for Grounding and Connection

These rituals can be woven into everyday caregiving:

- **Morning Greeting Ritual**
  Begin each day with the same phrase and gesture: "Good morning, beautiful," while opening the curtains and placing their favorite blanket around their shoulders.

- **Afternoon Tea or Snack Time**
  Serve tea in the same cup or use a special napkin each day. Play the same soft music in the background. This becomes a daily oasis.

- **Evening Wind-Down**
  Light a candle, rub lavender lotion on their hands, and sit quietly together for five minutes. Repeat the same lullaby, prayer, or poem to close the day.

- **Gratitude Hand-Holding**
  At mealtimes, hold hands and each say (or simply feel) something you're thankful for. Even silence, held together, can be a ritual of gratitude.

Weekly or Monthly Joy Traditions

Create consistent rhythms that offer something to look forward to:

- **Music Mondays**
  Play a specific playlist each Monday afternoon. Include songs from their youth or calming instrumental favorites. Maybe add dancing or chair movement.

- **Story Saturdays**
  Choose a short poem or picture book to read aloud. No need for comprehension—let tone and rhythm be the gift.

- **Nature Walk Fridays**
  Take a short walk outside each week, even just to the porch or garden. Point out leaves, clouds, birds. Make it a ritual of shared wonder.

- **Creative Rituals**
  Finger paint. Fold paper. Arrange flowers. Repeat the same activity weekly, not to build skills—but to invite play and connection.

Adapted Holiday Rituals

Holidays can be painful reminders of what's changed. But they can also be beautifully reimagined:

- **Simplify the Season**
  Instead of large family gatherings, have smaller, quieter visits. Dim the lights. Choose one carol instead of a whole concert. Let the ritual be the *feeling*, not the event.

- **Honor Without Expectation**
  Place a candle by a photo of a loved one who has passed. Don't ask them to remember—just hold space.

- **Involve the Senses**
  Bake a familiar treat. Light a holiday-scented candle. Wrap and unwrap a small, soft gift. These tangible cues spark emotional memory.

- **Intergenerational Joy**
  Invite grandchildren to perform a simple song or bring handmade cards. Repetition and rhythm create cross-generational rituals that bypass memory and go straight to the heart.

Inventing New Rituals from the Present Moment

You don't need a reason or a tradition to start a ritual. Look for moments of natural resonance, then name and repeat them.

Examples:

- **"Blue Mug Time"** – Every afternoon, you sit with tea in a blue mug. Over time, the mug itself becomes a signal for calm connection.

- **"Sock Parade"** – Each morning, your loved one picks silly socks. You both cheer when they're on.

- **"Sunset Sitting"** – You watch the sun go down together, without needing to speak.

Rituals don't have to be elaborate. They simply need to be *repeated with love*.

The Caregiver's Personal Rituals

While creating rituals for your loved one is powerful, **caregivers need rituals too**—to stay grounded, nourished, and emotionally balanced.

Try:

- **Start-of-Day Grounding**
  Before waking your loved one, place your hand on your heart and say, "I am here. I am enough. This moment matters."

- **Nightly Letting Go**
  After bedtime, light a candle and release the day. Say aloud or silently, "What's done is done. I did my best. Tomorrow is a new day."

- **Weekly Reset**
  Choose one day per week to step away, even briefly. Walk in nature, call a friend, write, or sit in stillness. Repeat weekly without fail.

- **Gratitude Journal**
  Keep a simple log: one moment of joy, one thing you handled with grace, one thing you're proud of.

These rituals affirm that *you*, too, are worthy of care.

Creating Rituals with Family and Friends

Rituals can also become **shared commitments** among the care circle. Try:

- **Photo Message Chain**
  Family members take turns sending a daily or weekly photo of their day. Print and display them as part of a visual ritual for your loved one.

- **Memory Night**
  Once a month, family gathers to share memories aloud—not to test the person with dementia, but to hold collective remembering.

- **Ritual Calls**
  A grandchild calls every Wednesday to sing a song or tell a joke. The call may not be remembered—but the joy lands each time.

In Closing

When memory fades, ritual remains.

In a world where past and future feel slippery, rituals say: *Here is something you can count on. Here is a rhythm we can share. Here is a moment that matters.*

You don't need to preserve every tradition. You don't need to recreate the past.
You only need to be present enough to notice what feels good, and *do it again with intention.*

These small acts, repeated with love, become sacred.
They become anchors.
They become **rituals of joy**.

In the next chapter, we'll go deeper into non-verbal connection. How can we communicate beyond language—through music, touch, movement, and presence? What does it mean to truly "listen" when words are no longer available?

Chapter 13: Language Without Words – Music, Touch, and Intuition

Communicating When Language Fades

As Alzheimer's and other forms of dementia progress, spoken language often slips away. Words get tangled. Sentences trail off. Questions repeat endlessly—or stop altogether. This loss can be profoundly painful, especially in relationships built on conversation, storytelling, and verbal affirmation.

But here's the truth: **connection doesn't end when words do.**

In fact, some of the deepest, most meaningful moments between caregivers and loved ones happen in silence—in a gesture, a glance, a hum, a heartbeat shared. As verbal language recedes, another kind of communication emerges—**the language of the body, the senses, and the soul.**

In this chapter, we'll explore how to tune into and expand this silent language. Through music, touch, movement, and emotional intuition, we can continue—and even deepen—our relationships, discovering that connection does not depend on words. It depends on presence.

The Myth That Communication = Speech

Western culture privileges verbal language. We define intelligence, emotional health, and even personhood through the ability to speak, explain, and respond coherently. When language fades, it's often assumed that the person is "gone," or that meaningful communication is no longer possible.

But this is a **cultural myth**, not a biological truth.

From infancy to the end of life, human beings rely on **non-verbal communication**—tone of voice, facial expression, eye contact, physical proximity, and movement. In fact, studies show that more than 70% of human communication is non-verbal.

People with dementia often become more attuned to this non-verbal landscape as verbal language fades. They may respond more to tone than to meaning, more to rhythm than to syntax. They may pick up on your emotions long before your words land.

If we adjust to this new language, we can still speak volumes.

Music: Memory's Secret Passageway

Music is often described as the last language to go. Long after a person has stopped speaking or recognizing loved ones, they may still:

- Tap a rhythm on their lap

- Hum or sing familiar songs

- Smile at the opening notes of a favorite melody

- Cry or laugh in response to a song from their youth

This is because music bypasses the language centers of the brain and accesses **emotion and long-term memory** through other neural pathways.

Music becomes a **bridge**—to joy, to self, to shared moments.

How to Use Music Intentionally:

- **Create a Personal Playlist**
  Include songs from their adolescence or young adulthood—the period often most deeply encoded in long-term memory.

- **Sing Together**
Singing with them, even off-key, can create a shared rhythm and deepen connection.

- **Use Instrumentals for Calm**
Soft piano or nature sounds can soothe during moments of anxiety or restlessness.

- **Match the Mood**
Uplifting music for mornings. Calming music for evening wind-down. Let music support their emotional rhythm.

- **Move Together**
Clap, sway, or dance in your chairs. Let the music animate both of you.

Touch: The Original Language

Before we speak, we are held. Before we write, we are rocked. Touch is the first language we learn—and often the last we forget.

People with memory loss may not recognize you by name, but they may still lean into your embrace. A gentle hand on the back or a stroke along the forearm can communicate what words cannot: **"You are safe. You are loved. I am here."**

Forms of Healing Touch:

- **Hand-holding** – Simple, grounding, human.

- **Hair brushing** – Repetitive and soothing, often associated with care and intimacy.

- **Gentle massage** – Shoulders, hands, or feet. Use lotion with a calming scent like lavender.

- **Reassuring strokes** – Light pressure on the back or arm during distress can offer immediate comfort.

- **Palm-to-palm contact** – Sit quietly, palms touching. Let the silence speak.

Always approach touch slowly and with permission. Watch for cues of comfort or discomfort. Respect boundaries. What soothes one person may irritate another.

Movement: Expression Through the Body

As language declines, many people retain an instinctive connection to **rhythm and motion**. Dancing, walking, rocking, or even simple gestures become ways of participating in life and relationship.

Ideas for Movement-Based Connection:

- **Chair dancing** – Move arms together to a familiar song. Mirror their motions gently.

- **Walking side by side** – Even slow pacing in a hallway can be calming and connective.

- **Ball toss** – A soft ball passed back and forth creates interaction and rhythm.

- **Stretching together** – Guided gentle stretches can reconnect body awareness and ease restlessness.

- **Imitating gestures** – If your loved one starts tapping or moving their fingers, do it too. Let it become a shared rhythm.

Movement brings people into the **present moment**, grounding them in their bodies and the physical world.

Intuition: Listening Beyond Logic

When we stop relying on language, we begin to listen with new ears. We become more attuned to **emotion, energy, and instinct**. We stop asking, "What are they trying to say?" and start asking, "What do they feel? What do they need?"

This is **empathic listening**. It's not about decoding words—it's about tuning into presence.

Tips for Building Intuitive Listening:

- **Match their emotion, not their words.** If they say something cheerful with a confused expression, reflect their feeling, not their content.

- **Watch body language.** Tension in the shoulders, clenched hands, or fidgeting may indicate discomfort.

- **Use silence.** Don't rush to fill every gap. Let the space breathe.

- **Validate emotion first.** "You seem a little anxious right now. I'm here."

- **Trust your gut.** If you feel a shift in energy, respond to it gently. Your instincts are often correct.

Intuitive connection may feel subtle at first—but it grows with attention. It is deeply human.

Creating an Environment That Speaks

Beyond our interactions, the environment itself becomes a form of non-verbal communication. A well-designed space can say:

- "You are safe."

- "You are at home."

- "You matter here."

Environmental Language Strategies:

- **Familiar objects:** Photos, blankets, or knick-knacks from earlier years provide emotional anchoring.

- **Color cues:** Warm, soft colors can soothe. Harsh contrasts can overstimulate.

- **Natural light:** Sunlight improves mood and regulates circadian rhythms.

- **Soundscapes:** Gentle background sounds—birds, ocean waves, soft music—can provide comfort.

- **Scent rituals:** Use familiar smells (fresh bread, lavender, lemon) to evoke memory or create calm.

The goal is not stimulation, but **attunement**—creating an environment that feels emotionally readable, stable, and kind.

When Silence Speaks

There will be moments when no words are spoken. Perhaps no gestures are made. Just silence.

Don't rush to fill it.

Sit beside them. Breathe with them. Let your presence be enough.

Sometimes the most profound love is **silent**, shared not in speech, but in being. In these moments, the noise of identity, time, and expectation falls away—and what's left is *pure presence*.

Practices for Non-Verbal Connection

1. **"Just One Song" Ritual**
   Choose one familiar song. Sing it, hum it, or play it daily—always at the same time. Let the consistency and melody create emotional memory.

2. **Mirror Movement**
   For 3–5 minutes, gently mirror their hand gestures, facial expressions, or posture. This creates non-verbal empathy and synchrony.

3. **Touch & Say**
   While offering physical care, pair each touch with a word: "Warm," "Soft," "Here," "Safe." Use your tone to soothe.

4. **Emotional Translation**
   When they say something confusing, respond not to the words, but the **emotion underneath**. "You're scared? I'm here." "You miss someone?"

5. **Stillness Practice**
   Once a day, sit quietly together for one minute. Hold their hand. Just breathe. No talking. Let silence hold the space.

In Closing

When words disappear, we do not lose connection—we find a new one.
When names are forgotten, feelings remain.
When stories fade, presence endures.

Language is beautiful, but it is not the only way we know each other. Through rhythm, touch, music, and intuition, we continue to love—and be loved.

In the silence, a new language is born.
One that does not require memory.
Only presence.

Only heart.

In the next chapter, we'll explore what it means to see aging and cognitive decline not as diminishing, but as a form of *ascension*—a spiritual movement beyond ego, into something vaster. Can we honor this stage of life as a sacred unfolding?

Chapter 14: Aging as Ascension – The Soul Beyond Selfhood

Reframing Cognitive Decline as a Spiritual Unfolding

There is a quiet reverence we often reserve for birth—a sacred awe that surrounds new life entering the world. The baby doesn't speak, doesn't remember, doesn't know itself in the way adults do. And yet we gaze upon it with profound wonder, sensing something holy in its beingness.

What if we offered the same reverence to the other end of the human arc?

What if, instead of seeing aging and memory loss as decline, we saw them as **ascension**—a letting go of ego, of linear time, of the need to define and perform, in order to return to something deeper, more essential, more eternal?

In this chapter, we explore the idea that aging, and especially cognitive decline, may be a *spiritual unfolding* rather than simply a biological breakdown. While the Western world is steeped in narratives of deterioration, loss, and tragedy, other cultures and spiritual frameworks suggest something radically different: that the soul is rising even as the mind releases its hold on story.

Beyond Ego: Who Are We Without Our Roles?

In early adulthood and midlife, we build ourselves through roles and achievements. We become students, professionals, parents, partners. We collect identities like armor, shaping and reshaping them through memory, performance, and purpose.

But these roles, however meaningful, are temporary. They are garments worn by the self—not the self itself.

When Alzheimer's begins to loosen the threads of those roles—forgetting names, duties, even lifelong passions—it can feel devastating. Yet underneath the grief, something ancient is happening: **the dismantling of ego**.

From a spiritual perspective, the ego is not our essence. It's our interface with the world. It organizes, plans, protects, and identifies—but it is not the soul.

And so, as memory fades and roles dissolve, what remains is not nothing. What remains is **being**. Presence. The person in their most elemental state—free from ambition, self-narration, or image-management.

Some mystics would say: what remains is *truth*.

Mystical Teachings on Surrender and Loss of Self

Throughout spiritual traditions, the loss of self is not seen as a failure. It is the goal.

- **Buddhism** speaks of *anatta*—the "no-self"—as the path to enlightenment. Releasing attachment to identity and thought is a core practice of awakening.

- **Christian mystics** like St. John of the Cross spoke of "the dark night of the soul" as a necessary passage in which the self is stripped of all familiar ground—so that union with God becomes possible.

- **Sufi poets** like Rumi wrote of forgetting the self to merge with the Beloved:

"Be like a tree and let the dead leaves drop."

- **Taoism** speaks of returning to the source—not through knowledge, but through simplicity, flow, and surrender.

What if dementia—far from a disorder to be fought—is an unintentional but profound enactment of these teachings?

What if the person forgetting names and places is actually **returning**—not to childhood, but to the soul?

From Doing to Being

In a society obsessed with doing, the person with dementia becomes a mirror. They no longer produce in the ways we expect. They do not remember to strive. They don't plan or perform. They sit. They feel. They are.

This shift is often interpreted as regression.

But perhaps it is **ascension**.

As thought and language fade, the person becomes more attuned to the rhythms of life: light and dark, warmth and cold, music and silence, love and fear. Their presence, though "unproductive," begins to reveal another kind of intelligence—a *being intelligence*.

They do not do—they *are*.

And in this beingness, we are invited to slow down, to listen, to join them in the stillness.

The Caregiver as Witness to Ascension

To care for someone with dementia is to witness this transformation. And it requires a shift in your own consciousness. You are no longer supporting someone's rise through achievement or independence. You are accompanying them through *unbecoming*.

This is sacred work.

It is similar to midwifery—but for the other end of life. You are not restoring function. You are *holding space* as the person returns to essence.

This doesn't mean ignoring suffering or romanticizing decline. There are hard days. Painful days. But if you look closely, you may also see:

- A peace that comes when words are no longer needed.

- A childlike wonder in watching trees or touching water.

- A mysterious stillness in their eyes that feels like looking into the soul.

Your role is not to drag them back into old roles, but to honor the journey they're now on—a journey of release.

Signs of Spiritual Presence in Cognitive Absence

You might witness moments that don't make logical sense but carry a deep, resonant energy:

- A person who hasn't spoken in weeks suddenly says "thank you" or "I love you."

- A gaze that lingers and softens, as if seeing something beyond the room.

- A sudden burst of song, prayer, or poetry—unrehearsed, spontaneous, pure.

- Tears that arise for no clear reason, as though processing something beyond words.

These are not clinical phenomena alone. They may be glimpses of the soul speaking.

When we stop judging these moments as "delusions" or "symptoms," we begin to feel their sacred weight.

Reframing the End of the Story

Western culture frames the final chapters of life as diminishment—a winding down, a fading out.

But in spiritual traditions, the end of life is often the **climax**—the culmination of a soul's journey. Not a decline, but an ascent.

What if we reframed the dementia journey accordingly?

- Not: "She's losing everything."
  But: "She's shedding what no longer serves her."

- Not: "He doesn't know who he is anymore."
  But: "He's beyond the need to define himself."

- Not: "They're disappearing."
  But: "They're transforming."

Such reframing isn't a denial of loss—it's a reorientation toward meaning. It allows us to hold both: the pain of what is gone and the reverence for what is emerging.

Practices for Seeing the Soul

1. **Sacred Gaze**
   Spend five minutes simply looking into your loved one's eyes, with no agenda. Imagine you are looking into the eternal part of them—not the person you remember, but the soul that always was.

2. **Soul Language Journal**
   Each day, write down one non-verbal moment that felt sacred: a glance, a sigh, a gesture. Begin to build a vocabulary for soul presence.

3. **Anointing Touch**

   During caregiving tasks, treat the body with reverence. Wash their hands like a ritual. Comb their hair like a prayer.

4. **Breath Synchronization**

   Sit side-by-side. Align your breathing. Let the shared rhythm become a meditation—a reminder that presence doesn't need memory.

5. **Silent Witnessing**

   Each week, spend time with them without words. No music. No talking. Just be. Let the silence speak. Let the stillness deepen your connection.

In Closing

We are not our memories.
We are not our thoughts.
We are not our stories.

We are the awareness behind all of it.
We are presence.
We are soul.

As dementia strips away the outer layers of identity, something ineffable remains.
Something sacred.
Something eternal.

If we allow ourselves to see dementia not only as disappearance but as *ascension*, then we meet our loved ones not with fear, but with awe.

And in doing so, we begin our own ascent too—rising into a deeper understanding of what it means to love, to be, to surrender.

In the final chapter, we will explore how to carry all of this forward. How do we begin creating a culture that holds memory loss, aging, and caregiving with compassion, creativity, and reverence? What legacy do we leave when we walk the path of forgetting with grace?

Chapter 15: Creating a Culture of Compassionate Presence

Reimagining How We Hold Aging, Memory Loss, and Each Other

Throughout this book, we've journeyed together through the winding, intimate, and often mysterious landscape of memory loss. We've explored how to release old narratives of tragedy, find joy in the present, communicate beyond words, and meet both ourselves and our loved ones with tenderness and awe.

But this transformation—this sacred reframing—cannot remain solely in the private realm. If we are to truly shift the experience of Alzheimer's and dementia, it must ripple outward. It must shape **culture**.

We must ask:

What kind of world are we building for those who forget?
And what kind of world are we building for those who care?

In this final chapter, we envision a future where memory loss is no longer hidden in shame or isolation—but met with community, beauty, and love. Where care is not only a duty but a creative, collective act. Where we move from a culture of fear and denial to a culture of **compassionate presence**.

This is not an abstract ideal. It is a call to action.

The Culture We Inherit

In much of the Western world, aging is seen as a problem. Decline. Burden. Expense. Dementia, especially, is framed as a personal and societal tragedy—a narrative fueled by fear, misunderstanding, and disconnection.

Consider the dominant cultural messages:

- Memory is identity.

- Productivity equals worth.

- Aging must be resisted at all costs.

- Dementia is death-in-life.

These assumptions isolate the elderly. They exhaust caregivers. They generate stigma. They strip away dignity.

But culture is not fixed.
It is built—and it can be rebuilt.

Rewriting the Collective Story

We need new stories. Not to sugarcoat memory loss, but to expand the lens.

We need to tell stories that:

- Celebrate **presence** over productivity.

- Highlight **caregiving** as spiritual and creative work.

- Show people with dementia as *beings of worth*, not merely patients.

- Reflect the full spectrum of the journey—not just the sorrow, but the joy, the connection, the beauty.

These stories can come from:

- **Caregivers' voices** sharing their moments of grace.

- **People living with dementia** telling their truth in the early stages.

- **Artists, filmmakers, and writers** crafting new, compassionate portrayals.

- **Families and communities** honoring their elders through presence, not pity.

We must flood the culture with examples of love that adapts, connection that transcends cognition, and dignity that does not depend on memory.

Building Dementia-Inclusive Communities

Compassionate presence isn't just a mindset—it's a design principle. What would it look like to create communities where people with memory loss are not just tolerated, but *welcomed*, supported, and even celebrated?

Examples of What's Possible:

- **Dementia-friendly public spaces**: Parks, libraries, cafes, and stores designed with clear signage, calm acoustics, sensory cues, and staff training.

- **Intergenerational programs**: Children spending time in eldercare centers, learning empathy and non-verbal communication through play and art.

- **Memory cafés**: Monthly gatherings where people with dementia and their families come together to enjoy music, laughter, and connection without judgment.

- **Training for first responders and service workers**: Helping everyone from paramedics to bank tellers respond with compassion and patience to those who may be confused.

- **Creative arts programs**: Music, dance, painting, and storytelling sessions that invite expression beyond words.

- **Neighborhood care circles**: Local volunteers offering respite for caregivers, companionship for elders, and the kind of support that prevents isolation.

Honoring Caregivers as Cultural Stewards

In a culture of compassionate presence, **caregivers are not invisible**.

They are not sidelined, shamed, or asked to carry impossible burdens alone. They are honored as spiritual companions, emotional first responders, and community anchors.

This requires:

- **Access to resources**: Affordable home care, respite services, financial support.

- **Mental health care**: Therapy, counseling, support groups that see caregiving not just as logistics, but as emotional labor.

- **Rituals of recognition**: Community acknowledgments of caregivers—whether through art, ceremony, storytelling, or shared meals.

Caregivers are not "doing it wrong" when they feel tired, sad, or lost. In fact, they are doing the most human work there is: loving someone through transformation.

Creating New Rituals of Cultural Reverence

Every culture has rituals for major transitions—birth, marriage, death. But few have rituals for the long, slow shift of memory loss. We need new rites—not only to mark loss, but to **celebrate presence**.

Imagine:

- **Letting Go Ceremonies**: A gathering where a family collectively acknowledges that their loved one no longer remembers names, and blesses the journey forward in the present.

- **Gratitude Altars**: A small corner of the home with candles, flowers, or objects that represent moments of connection, joy, and resilience in the dementia journey.

- **Caregiver Sabbaths**: A monthly day of rest, reflection, and reconnection—supported by community volunteers.

- **Storytelling Vigils**: A shared space where people gather to tell stories *to* their loved one, not expecting recognition, but offering presence.

These rituals don't erase grief—but they give it form. They remind us: we are not alone. We are part of something sacred and shared.

Educating the Next Generation

To change the culture, we must change how future generations understand aging.

Let children see dementia not as a loss of humanity, but a shift in how humanity is expressed. Let teens volunteer in eldercare centers. Let college students explore caregiving not just in health sciences, but in philosophy, ethics, and art.

Let love across generations be modeled early—and often.

When young people learn that presence is enough, that love does not depend on recognition, they carry that lesson forward into how they care for others—and themselves.

The Legacy of Compassionate Presence

What is the legacy of walking through memory loss with presence and love?

It is not just about helping one person die well.
It is about helping many people **live well**—even through forgetting.

It is about:

- A granddaughter who learns to love her grandmother through song, not speech.

- A son who stops asking his father to remember—and starts holding his hand.

- A community that replaces shame with shared care.

- A culture that dares to slow down and witness the sacredness of being.

You—yes, *you*—who have walked this path with presence, who have read these pages with your heart open, are already helping to build this culture.

One choice at a time. One moment of softness at a time. One surrender at a time.

In Closing

Memory is a beautiful thread in the tapestry of life—but it is not the only one.

Even as the thread of memory frays, others remain: touch, music, intuition, laughter, presence, soul.

We can mourn what is lost *and* celebrate what remains.

We can care not by clinging, but by releasing.

We can love not through memory, but through *presence*.

Let this be the culture we co-create.
A culture of compassionate presence.
A culture where forgetting is not exile—but transformation.
A culture where no one walks the path alone.

Thank you for walking this path with me. May you carry this vision forward—with courage, with gentleness, and with the deep knowing that love, in its truest form, is never forgotten.

The End
But also, the beginning.

Bibliography

Books & Memoirs

- Alzheimer's Association. (2024). *2024 Alzheimer's Disease Facts and Figures.* Alzheimer's & Dementia, 20(3), 1–140.

- Byock, Ira. (2012). *The Best Care Possible: A Physician's Quest to Transform Care Through the End of Life.* Avery.

- Cohen, Gene D. (2005). *The Mature Mind: The Positive Power of the Aging Brain.* Basic Books.

- Doidge, Norman. (2007). *The Brain That Changes Itself: Stories of Personal Triumph from the Frontiers of Brain Science.* Viking.

- Gawande, Atul. (2014). *Being Mortal: Medicine and What Matters in the End.* Metropolitan Books.

- Halpern, Megan Carnarius. (2015). *A Deeper Perspective on Alzheimer's and Other Dementias: Practical Tools with Spiritual Insights.* Findhorn Press.

- Hepworth, David. (2015). *Caregiving: A Shared Journey.* Open Heart Press.

- Killick, John & Allan, Kate. (2001). *Communication and the Care of People with Dementia.* Open University Press.

- Kitwood, Tom. (1997). *Dementia Reconsidered: The Person Comes First.* Open University Press.

- McFarlane, Graham Stokes. (2008). *And Still the Music Plays: Stories of People with Dementia.* Hawker Publications.

- McLean, Beth. (2021). *Holding Time: Aging With Grace and Letting Go of the Past.* Spiritwell Press.

- Powers, Beth. (2018). *Dancing with Dementia: My Story of Living Positively with Dementia.* Jessica Kingsley Publishers.

- Thomas, Bill. (2004). *What Are Old People For? How Elders Will Save the World.* VanderWyk & Burnham.

Journal Articles and Reports

- Kontos, Pia. (2005). "Embodied Selfhood in Alzheimer's Disease: Rethinking Person-Centred Care." *Dementia*, 4(4), 553–570.

- Sabat, Steven R. (2001). *The Experience of Alzheimer's Disease: Life Through a Tangled Veil.* Blackwell Publishers.

- Zeisel, John. (2009). "I'm Still Here: A New Philosophy of Alzheimer's Care." *American Journal of Alzheimer's Disease & Other Dementias*, 24(1), 1–10.

Spiritual and Cultural Texts

- Chödrön, Pema. (1997). *When Things Fall Apart: Heart Advice for Difficult Times.* Shambhala.

- Rumi, Jalal al-Din. (2004). *The Essential Rumi* (Trans. Coleman Barks). HarperOne.

- Hanh, Thich Nhat. (1992). *Peace Is Every Step: The Path of Mindfulness in Everyday Life.* Bantam.

- Tutu, Desmond & Tutu, Mpho. (2014). *The Book of Forgiving: The Fourfold Path for Healing Ourselves and Our World.* HarperOne.

- Tolle, Eckhart. (1999). *The Power of Now: A Guide to Spiritual Enlightenment.* New World Library.

Cultural and Cross-Traditional Sources

- Cohen, Lawrence. (1993). "Culture, Disease, and Memory: The 'Other' Alzheimer's." *Cultural Anthropology*, 8(1), 20–40.

- Kitwood, Tom. (1993). "Toward a Theory of Dementia Care: The Interpersonal Process." *Ageing and Society*, 13(1), 51–67.

- Taylor, James. (2008). "Ubuntu and the Ethics of Care." *Journal of Human Development and Capabilities*, 9(1), 27–45.

- Yeo, G., & Gallagher-Thompson, D. (2006). *Ethnic and Cultural Diversity in Dementia Care: A Review of Recent Literature.* Alzheimer's Association.

Web and Multimedia Resources

- Alzheimer's Society UK. (n.d.). *Dementia-Friendly Communities.* https://www.alzheimers.org.uk

- Dementia Alliance International. (n.d.). *Voices of People Living with Dementia.* https://www.dementiaallianceinternational.org

- Music & Memory Organization. (n.d.). *How Music Helps People with Dementia.* https://www.musicandmemory.org

- The Eden Alternative. (n.d.). *Reimagining Elder Care.* https://www.edenalt.org

Interviews, Observations & Lived Experience

Many of the reflections and narratives in this book are also informed by:

- Personal interviews with caregivers and care workers (2020–2024)

- Observations in dementia-friendly community programs and music therapy sessions

- Conversations with persons living with early-onset Alzheimer's and their families

- Insights from online support communities and forums for caregivers

---

Note to the Reader

This bibliography is a reflection of sources that inspired the philosophical, practical, and cultural reframing of memory loss found in this book. It honors both the scholarship and the *lived experience* that continue to guide a more compassionate and joyful approach to the dementia journey.

Glossary

Alzheimer's Disease

A progressive, degenerative brain disorder that gradually destroys memory, thinking skills, and the ability to carry out everyday tasks. It is the most common cause of dementia in older adults.

Ascension (Spiritual)

In this book's context, "ascension" refers to a spiritual rising or unfolding—a process of moving beyond the ego or surface identity to return to one's essential or soul-based self.

Anatta (No-Self)

A central concept in Buddhist philosophy meaning "not-self." It refers to the idea that the self is not a fixed, permanent entity but a collection of ever-changing physical and mental phenomena.

Autobiographical Memory

A type of long-term memory that involves recollection of personal experiences, including time, place, and emotions—often used to construct identity and self-narrative.

Caregiver (or Care Partner)

A person who provides physical, emotional, or practical support to someone who can no longer fully care for themselves. In the dementia context, caregivers often help with daily tasks, emotional reassurance, and presence.

Cognitive Decline

A term referring to the gradual loss of cognitive abilities such as memory, reasoning, language, and executive function, often associated with aging or neurodegenerative diseases.

Compassionate Presence

A central theme of the book, referring to the practice of being fully present with someone—especially someone experiencing memory loss—with empathy, acceptance, and non-judgment.

Dementia

An umbrella term for a group of symptoms affecting memory, thinking, behavior, and emotion. Alzheimer's is the most common type. Dementia is not a normal part of aging.

Emotional Memory

A form of implicit memory that allows people to retain and respond to feelings, even when explicit memories (events, people, timelines) are lost.

Essence-Based Love

A kind of love that exists beyond memory, roles, or recognition. It is based in presence, emotional attunement, and intuitive connection.

Ego (Psychological/Spiritual)

In psychology, the ego refers to the conscious self, identity, and self-image. In spiritual contexts, ego often refers to the constructed self or persona that separates us from deeper being or unity.

Limbic System

A complex set of brain structures involved in emotion, behavior, and long-term memory. It remains relatively intact in the earlier stages of dementia, allowing emotional connection even when memory fades.

Mirror Neurons

Brain cells that allow us to empathize and reflect the actions and emotions of others. These are involved in non-verbal connection, such as mirroring gestures or facial expressions.

Moment-Based Relationship

A relationship grounded in present-moment experience rather than shared history or verbal recall. These relationships emphasize emotional presence over narrative continuity.

Music Therapy

A clinical and evidence-based use of music interventions—such as listening, singing, or playing instruments—to accomplish personalized therapeutic goals, especially useful in dementia care.

Non-Verbal Communication

Conveying meaning without words, through facial expressions, gestures, tone of voice, touch, posture, and body movement. This becomes primary in later stages of memory loss.

Person-Centered Care

An approach to care that respects and values the individual as a whole person, with needs, preferences, and dignity—regardless of cognitive ability.

Presence

A state of being fully engaged, aware, and emotionally available in the current moment. Presence is often more valuable than memory in connecting with people who have dementia.

Radical Acceptance

A therapeutic concept that involves fully acknowledging reality as it is—without resistance, judgment, or denial. In caregiving, it allows for greater peace and connection.

Repetition Ritual

A calming or joyful activity repeated at regular intervals (daily, weekly) that creates emotional safety and connection, even when the person cannot recall past instances.

Ritual

A symbolic act or repeated sequence that creates meaning, emotional resonance, and connection. In dementia care, rituals can replace complex traditions and anchor the present.

Surrender (Spiritual/Emotional)

The intentional release of control, expectation, or resistance. In this context, surrender means accepting the changes that dementia brings and meeting them with love, rather than fear.

Ubuntu

A Southern African philosophy emphasizing human interconnectedness: *"I am because we are."* It values collective care and sees personhood as rooted in community.

Validation Therapy

A therapeutic approach that encourages accepting the reality and emotions of people with dementia, rather than correcting or challenging their perceptions.

Verbal Language Decline

A symptom of dementia involving difficulty in finding words, forming sentences, or understanding speech. This often requires new, non-verbal ways of relating.

Witnessing (Spiritual Practice)

Being present with another person without judgment or the need to fix—holding space for their reality and experience. This becomes a sacred role in caregiving.

Yes, And... (Improv Principle)

A technique borrowed from improvisational theater where one accepts and builds on what another person says. In dementia care, it helps create playful, validating interactions rather than correction or resistance.